Governance, democracy and ethics in crisis-decision-making

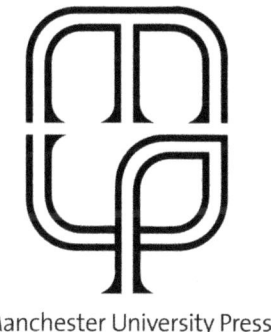

Manchester University Press

Governance, democracy and ethics in crisis-decision-making

The pandemic and beyond

Edited by

Caroline Redhead and Melanie Smallman

MANCHESTER UNIVERSITY PRESS

Copyright © Manchester University Press 2024

While copyright in the volume as a whole is vested in Manchester University Press, copyright in individual chapters belongs to their respective authors, and no chapter may be reproduced wholly or in part without the express permission in writing of both author and publisher.

An electronic version has been made freely available under a Creative Commons (CC BY) licence, which permits commercial use, distribution and reproduction provided the author(s) and Manchester University Press are fully cited. Details of the licence can be viewed at https://creativecommons.org/licenses/by/4.0/

This work was supported by the Arts and Humanities Research Council.

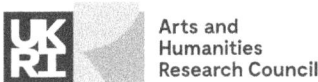

Published by Manchester University Press
Oxford Road, Manchester, M13 9PL

www.manchesteruniversitypress.co.uk

British Library Cataloguing-in-Publication Data
A catalogue record for this book is available from the British Library

ISBN 978 1 5261 8004 9 hardback

First published 2024

The publisher has no responsibility for the persistence or accuracy of URLs for any external or third-party internet websites referred to in this book, and does not guarantee that any content on such websites is, or will remain, accurate or appropriate.

Typeset by Newgen Publishing UK

Contents

Series preface: The pandemic and beyond – Pascale Aebischer, Fred Cooper, Des Fitzgerald, Karen Gray, Caroline Redhead, Melanie Smallman and Victoria Tischler — vii
List of figures and tables — xxv
Contributors — xxvi
Acknowledgements — xxx

Introduction – Melanie Smallman and Caroline Redhead — 1

1 The epidemic as a life-event: epidemicity and epidemic form – Lina Minou, James Wilson and Daniel Herron — 12
2 Relationships were a casualty when pandemic ethics and everyday clinical ethics collided – Caroline Redhead, Anna Chiumento, Sara Fovargue, Heather Draper and Lucy Frith — 29
3 Evaluating post-pandemic plans for social care data infrastructures – Cian O'Donovan — 54
4 Data ethics in an emergency – Melanie Smallman, Cian O'Donovan, James Wilson and Jack Hume — 77
5 Data-driven decision-making beyond COVID-19: incorporating the voice of the child – Claire Bessant and Rachel Allsopp — 94
6 Where are publics in pandemic public policy? – Jamie Webb and Kiran Kaur Manku — 124

7 From a crisis of confidence towards confidence in a crisis: what can we learn about the pandemic's impact on democracy? – Reema Patel 150

8 Accountability, transparency and good governance: the WHO's decision-making during an emergency – Harry Upton, Abbie-Rose Hampton and Mark Eccleston-Turner 172

Index 191

Series preface: The pandemic and beyond

Pascale Aebischer, Fred Cooper, Des Fitzgerald, Karen Gray, Caroline Redhead, Melanie Smallman and Victoria Tischler

In the first days of 2020, the coronavirus (COVID-19) pandemic began to spread across the globe. It prompted a concerted international research effort which set out to understand not just the workings of the virus, but the ways that we responded to, lived and died with it. This led to a significant body of work being produced at speed, in which arts and humanities played a crucial role. In the UK, *The Pandemic and Beyond: The Arts and Humanities Contribution to Covid Research and Recovery* was established by the Arts and Humanities Research Council (AHRC) early in 2021 to coordinate this research effort.[1] Over the span of two years, *The Pandemic and Beyond* grew into a virtual hub that enabled over seventy COVID-19 research teams funded by the AHRC to meet, exchange ideas and work together to ensure that their research would make a difference on the ground.[2]

This series is a legacy of this collaboration and bears witness to an extraordinary period, in which arts and humanities research became an integral part of the UK's research response to an emergency, leading to tangible changes in the role, purpose and methods of the arts and humanities, and laying important human foundations for recovery. It is divided into four volumes, each corresponding to four research clusters co-produced during the coordination process. A first group focused on working with professionals and policymakers in the creative industries to investigate the existential struggles of creative workers and organisations impacted by the ban on live in-person performance, and to devise new ways of connecting people through live arts while trying to build more inclusive and sustainable industry structures. A second set of research teams connected arts and creative practitioners with cultural and community organisations, as well as care settings, with whom they worked to alleviate the social and mental health impacts of public health restrictions. These projects drew on arts- and nature-based activities to forge pathways for improving mental and physical health for individuals and communities. A third cluster examined the informational and epistemic experience of a pandemic that was a whirlwind of often deeply confusing and contested data. Artists, designers and linguists explored design solutions and devised how public health messages could be formulated so that they would reach the communities most severely affected by the spread of the virus. A final group of researchers concentrated on scrutinising legislation and guidance issued in haste, and grappled with thorny questions of rights and responsibilities, seeking to underpin developing scientific understanding with values-based frameworks that offered a more nuanced approach to balancing risks and benefits.

The richness of this research portfolio stems not only from its breadth but also from the ingenuity of the teams involved, members of which rapidly applied their expertise and creativity to a problem few had foreseen, working with communities whose vulnerabilities and prior marginalisation had been exacerbated disproportionately by the pandemic (Ryan, 2022: 198). What was initially perceived principally as a public health crisis was impacting on the population in myriad ways that branched well beyond physical health; encompassing mental health, but also social cohesion, cross-generational justice, trust in governance, and economic distress. Looking back over the first few years of the pandemic, the authors of a report for the Higher Education Policy Institute (HEPI) conclude that the 'pandemic was a watershed moment for the Humanities because the importance of the variety and quality of individual human experience rose to the surface in our collective re-evaluation of priorities' (Thain et al., 2023: 13). Arts and humanities research concentrated on the human impacts of the crises that intersected in this moment, working to resolve them, mitigate harms and examine some of the most fundamental human questions across macro and micro crisis contexts, from the national and international to the local and hyper-local. As these volumes show, this work was characterised by cross-fertilisation between disciplines and an emphasis on partnership working. It featured collaboration; between academic and public institutions, but also, notably, with community groups and frontline organisations, such as those representing health and social care. Collaborations also extended to industry, and regional, sectoral and national policymakers. We know from analysis of surveys of those involved in *Pandemic and Beyond* research that for many this involved drawing on existing relationships, which deepened and strengthened as the fluctuations of the pandemic necessitated constant dialogue and increased accountability on all sides (Aebischer et al., 2022: 26–29). For others, the pandemic resulted in potentially fruitful new connections, and the promise of further research, work that continues to be relevant and have impacts on policy and practice.

All of this required new ways of working, and the ability to reconcile the theoretically conceptualised and deliberative methodologies associated with humanities research, which often take years to mature into publication, with quick and direct application, which often left little scope for fine calibration and reflective writing. The temporal demand for research outputs, and their new or altered audiences, exerted intense and immediate demands on researchers. Policymakers expressed an appetite for actionable findings to support decision-making, and frontline workers, while exhausted and short of time and resources, were desperate for support; research, in consequence, was predominantly pragmatic and focused on solutions. This meant a sometimes uneasy pivot to new ways of working and new modalities and timescales for doing and sharing work. Researchers did not always find it easy to reach those for whom their findings might have been most relevant, but many published policy briefings or held private meetings to share their insights and recommendations with potential user groups. Some projects embedded researchers within policy or service delivery organisations, narrowing the gap between research and practice still further. Work was often cyclical or iterative, with results shared earlier and more frequently, for example through pre-prints or the release of preliminary findings; if not a direct prerequisite for funding, the word 'rapid' in the UK Research and Innovation (UKRI) COVID-19 call certainly implied that researchers had to reconsider how and when in the life cycle of a project potentially significant knowledge was shared. There was a flowering of online engagement and dissemination as research was translated into a rich variety of deeply practical resources. These included frameworks for action, advice for public health messaging, interventions that responded to real-time problems such as the isolation of residents and staff in care homes or the design of personal protective equipment (PPE), and co-producing guidance for employers of artists performing in digital live shows from their homes.

As *Pandemic and Beyond* researchers explored the dynamic nature of individual and collective experiences of the pandemic, they also demonstrated a particular sensitivity to those for whom its effects have been felt unequally, and for whom suffering has been most profound. Readers will find this concern consistently exemplified throughout these volumes. Indeed, our brief to the authors in this series invited them to create a space where those voices could be part of the conversation. Such work was by no means easy to do. It was ethically complex, requiring heightened reflexivity and cultural competency. It was complicated by the requirements for social distancing and the need to prioritise the safety and wellbeing of both participants and researchers. As one research leader put it: 'you cannot build diversity into a project from scratch under these conditions' (Aebischer et al., 2022: 27).

Carrying out research during a pandemic necessitated innovation and adaptation at all levels. This is reflected in the research methods adopted: mixed, interdisciplinary and often participatory or arts-based, with projects bringing immediate benefits to participants and communities even as policymakers were targeted with written work. In many of the projects, more reflective and long-form modes of writing were either not part of the research design or postponed to a later date, to allow for retrospective analysis and evaluation. Meanwhile, the nascent field of arts and health was propelled to the foreground by the pandemic. A growing evidence base demonstrates the importance of multiple artistic modalities (including music, visual art, poetry and drama) in supporting health and wellbeing for a range of physical and mental health conditions. In these contexts, research by *Pandemic and Beyond* teams was able to highlight the vital role of artistic and creative practice through exposing the dangerousness of working conditions for frontline staff, including for the predominantly female workforce in social care settings. Arts-based projects were able to offer practical tools and emotional support for care workers, while helping to alleviate the isolation that many felt when confined to their homes by re-creating artistic activities that were delivered via post, online or outdoors. With remarkable speed, researchers working with arts and cultural providers pivoted to developing suitable resources and freely shared their work with collaborators and user groups.

At times, however, things moved frustratingly slowly, while structures around the research (including university recruitment, facilities, ethics and funding) creaked and failed to keep up; at other times, the most fundamental changes and compromises to research design had to be made at speed, to respond to events as they happened. When this research was at its best, there were refreshingly democratic opportunities for everyone involved to learn and apply new skills and take on new responsibilities. At their worst, however, the conditions in which research was conducted during the pandemic replicated existing structural problems in the academy. A great deal of the work was done by early career researchers on short-term contracts, for example, and researchers found themselves giving more than their contracted hours to this work, alongside their commitments to delivering newly remote or hybrid teaching, often while caring for home-schooled children or dealing with the impacts of the pandemic on their own networks and home environments. While it was often deeply rewarding, many researchers, like others in the population generally, found the lack of a distinction between home, work and the stresses of pandemic life difficult to negotiate. Remote working proved methodologically, physically and mentally challenging. However, as these chapters demonstrate so clearly, it led to the rapid creation and deployment of new tools and technologies for data collection, analysis and collaboration. These, in turn, are exerting pressure on funders and policymakers in UK Higher Education to adapt their frameworks to recognise the value and complexity of this type of crisis- and solutions-oriented collaborative response in arts and humanities research.

The work presented in this series as a distinctive and coherent portfolio is, of course, just part of a much wider programme of research to mitigate the effects of the pandemic and to address the COVID-19 emergency that was funded through UKRI.[3] While the projects within the *Pandemic and Beyond* portfolio were all designed, in line with the parameters of the original rapid-response funding call, to take a largely UK focus, a range of other projects and funding calls cast their gaze further afield. For some existing projects with an international focus, this 'created new opportunities for exploration of existing topics' that were exacerbated by the pandemic (Pirgova-Morgan, 2022: 27). Other schemes which are not represented in these volumes, for instance the UKRI Global Research Challenges/Newton Fund, brought together researchers in the UK and in low- and middle-income countries. More than forty such collaborative projects sought to gain insights and provide support during the pandemic, including projects aiming to improve engagement with COVID-19 public health messages to develop online psychological support through the arts in Rwanda; and to find ways of engaging vulnerable communities in Brazil on the consequences of the pandemic. This range of international projects is likely to offer an opportunity for further reflection, comparisons, dialogue and lessons in the future.

At the same time, we should not forget that despite the COVID-19 pandemic being, by definition, a global phenomenon, it has also been markedly culturally specific, local and hyper-local. Even in purely scientific terms, the identity of the virus itself has not been a global constant. Different strains and variants have emerged in different geographies and populations, and symptoms and morbidities have varied from country to country, creating very different patterns of disease across the world. Similarly, our responses to the pandemic and our standards of evidence and certainty – alongside modes of reasoning, ways of knowing and understanding – vary across cultural contexts, as we encounter different policymaking arrangements and civic communities. This is clear from the comparative work of the 'Lex Atlas' research in the *Pandemic and Beyond* portfolio, whose researchers examined dozens of countries' legal responses to the pandemic (King and Ferraz, 2021–23). Lessons learned in one country do not, therefore, translate cleanly to others.

Even within the UK, the response to COVID-19 was not uniformly governed or experienced. Nor did the disease spread evenly across the country. Time and time again, low-income households and communities, as well as groups with pre-existing vulnerabilities, felt the worst effects of both the disease and the measures put in place to protect the population. This pandemic was perhaps also one of the most challenging instances in which the arrangements for devolved administrations in Scotland, Wales and Northern Ireland,

and the powers of the Westminster Government to oversee or coordinate national responses, were put to the test, prompting comparative analysis of the different modes and mechanisms of parliamentary review across the UK. This was complemented by scrutiny of data-driven approaches to decision-making and research that probed ethical and human rights issues. A deep delve into the situation in the UK provides us with valuable insight into the state of the nation – as well as our collective experience of the COVID-19 pandemic – in the early twenty-first century.

While arts and humanities research on COVID-19 in the UK is ongoing, and many are now engaged in the more considered process of retrospective analysis and critique, this series, produced at the endpoint of the rapid-response funding period, does represent a significant milestone. As such, it offers an opportunity to reflect on the multiple temporalities and intersectional crises that have characterised the first two years of the pandemic, along with the wider epistemic structures and infrastructures at stake in the delivery of this research portfolio. While COVID-19 had a fairly temporally precise beginning in the final days of 2019, at least as a distinct viral emergency, and was formalised as a global emergency with the World Health Organization's (WHO) declaration of a pandemic on 11 March 2020, it can also be understood as, at least in part, the product of a deeper crisis in terms of anthropogenic climate change and how we interact with the non-human (Gupta et al., 2021). COVID-19 has been a profoundly transformative, rupturing crisis, with over two million dead in Europe alone (WHO, 2022b). Worldwide, anxiety and depression increased by 25 per cent (WHO, 2022a), and access to professional services was challenging; over 100 million lost their jobs (WEF, 2021), and while some accessed furlough and insurance payments, freelancers and those in the gig economy were often ineligible (Fowler, 2020). COVID-19 identified and shone a light on 'key workers', who were defined as those whose work was deemed essential during the pandemic and who often turned out to be poorly paid, socially marginalised and previously 'invisible'. These workers included healthcare professionals as well as bus drivers, food retailers, refuse collectors and care home staff. While healthcare staff were routinely celebrated in the UK, most notably through the 'clap for our carers' phenomenon, this was not accompanied by material changes in stagnant pay or harmful working conditions, and others – such as domiciliary workers in care homes with older people – remained largely invisible.

As the virus began to transform the ways that we live and die, it pulled a series of overlapping crises and temporalities into tension, muddying any clean imagining of a shared pandemic trajectory. When the UK government announced extensive restrictions to movement and social life in the spring of 2020, disability scholars and activists noted that many disabled people had effectively been in 'lockdown' for years (Shakespeare et al., 2021). Likewise, COVID-19 intersected with deep-seated inequalities in race and health, landing disproportionately among people who had their ability to resist the virus eroded by generations of structural racism, and who were knowingly figured as disposable and exposed to greater risk than their white counterparts (Qureshi et al., 2022). Whole groups of people, including frail older people and those with underlying health conditions, were disproportionately negatively impacted. Other long and slow disasters and matters of justice (such as poverty, burnout in healthcare workers, or our inability to sufficiently care for the old) further altered the temporal bounds of the pandemic and fragmented our experiences of pandemic time (Baraitser and Salisbury, 2020). For doctors, nurses, cleaners and porters in overstretched hospital departments, time sped up (often in catastrophic ways); for those who were shielding or placed on furlough, the opposite was frequently true.

Among this profound and intractable messiness, attempts to impose a temporal order on the pandemic have always done a particular kind of political work. Across the conception and execution of these four volumes, rates of infection, illness and death have been in considerable flux; the state of the pandemic at the date of publication is impossible to know as we write this introduction in early 2023. We do know, however, that pandemics rarely – if ever – cleanly end (Greene and Vargha, 2020). The overlapping contexts and crises detailed above also frame wildly divergent apprehensions and realities of risk. Any intimation that we are becoming 'post-pandemic' must be met with a question the arts and humanities are uniquely poised to ask: for whom? The bereaved, still shielding, sufferers from 'long COVID', carers and healthcare professionals, after all, will continue to live pandemic time in different ways (Callard and

Perego, 2021). One role of the arts and humanities amid this crisis is (or has been) to make and preserve *meaning* out of what has been experienced. In each of these volumes, 'rapid-response' arts and humanities work has had to navigate these slippery experiences of time. If many of our projects responded to the pandemic first in ways that were 'quick and dirty', acting to comprehend, forestall, or inform the present, the research assembled here is more inclined to the future, seeking to take a tentative and reflective step back from the immediacy of the pandemic while acknowledging its ongoing nature.

The format of the crisis-driven rapid-response call is itself an unusual approach to the organisation of arts and humanities research, with its distinctively longitudinal and reflective modes of relating to social problems. In one sense, this speedy deployment of the arts and humanities at a moment of crisis is welcome: it positions researchers within these disciplines as having skills that are critical for intervening in moments of emergency and lifts humanities research out of the epistemic position of providing commentary or representational analysis after the event. It thus refuses the disingenuous political position that cultural, literary, historical and theory-informed analysis is incompatible with the crisis resolution. Indeed, as this is a moment in which arts and humanities research is *itself* widely understood to be in crisis (see Thain et al., 2023), this instrumentalisation presents important new possibilities, and perhaps one or two pitfalls, for scholars within these disciplines. The assumption – implicit in the funding announcement – that research in the arts and humanities is already collaborative, engaged, pragmatic, problem-oriented, public-facing and interdisciplinary, an image which many in the humanities research community have been promoting for some years, often in the face of opposition from colleagues, is itself worthy of note.

This also follows a long-standing trend in which humanities research, whose structures have predominantly been based (somewhat stereotypically) on the model of a lone scholar, working diligently on their idiosyncratic topic over a period of years, is remade to resemble a more scientific model. Such a 'scientific model' notably involves the organisation of a project into research teams and work packages, the breaking down of disciplinary boundaries that are not methodologically salient, larger amounts of money being awarded to smaller numbers of research teams, the need to clearly articulate the public impact of research, and responsiveness to government and industry priorities. This trend has been clearly accelerated by the reorganisation of humanities research infrastructures during the COVID-19 pandemic, which, as we noted above, led to a much greater degree of collaboration, with several authors working remotely to write together, crossing institutional, geographical, disciplinary and hierarchical boundaries. The epistemic effects of such reorganisation have been real – and mixed. The organisation of research, after all, plays a large role in governing not just the type of writing possible in such circumstances, but also what research can and cannot be done. While the funding that framed the *Pandemic and Beyond* portfolio opened up many new possibilities for humanities researchers, it simultaneously foreclosed others. Scholars without a desire to work in teams, whose research did not need significant money or have clearly defined short- to medium-term impacts, will have struggled to contribute; a significant loss that mostly remains invisible. This portfolio showcases many new opportunities, but it also hides the opportunity costs – not only for humanities work directly on COVID-19, but for humanities research generally, as already scarce resources were poured into immediate responses to a single public health crisis.

In the context of a UK government research funding strategy which, as the March 2023 HEPI report notes, 'appears to downplay the position of the Arts and Humanities in the UK's ambition to become a "science superpower"' (Thain et al., 2023: 19), there is a wider political dimension to this, too. The COVID-19 crisis also coincided with a series of crises around Brexit, one of the most prominent of which concerned the possibility of the UK's participation in (or exclusion from) the EU's Horizon research programme. This created a context in which research was wielded openly as a token of national competitiveness, and international collaboration was reframed as a luxury that could be removed at a government's whim. While the UK focus of the *Pandemic and Beyond* research shielded this portfolio from some of these pressures, we nevertheless continuously faced the need to demonstrate, in a political climate ill-disposed to critical humanities thinking, the relevance, success, impact or transformational potential of this body of research. Against this backdrop, it was often tempting to frame our work to make it align with (party) political slogans such as 'build back better' or 'levelling up' to demonstrate a willingness to engage with political priorities. The need to establish such 'synergies' is now a common and perhaps unavoidable feature of research coordination and curation efforts such as that of *Pandemic and Beyond*. Indeed, the research we share through these volumes should also be understood in the context of a wider, global attack on the humanities, whether departmental closures in the United Kingdom, the driver for teaching efficiencies in Denmark, or legislative attacks in countries such as Hungary and the United States. The quick pivot to rapid-response work on COVID-19 is both an affirmative rebuttal to such attacks (our work is indeed both important and useful) *and* a frank recognition of how successful they have been (our work is only viable to the extent that we can successfully position it as both important and useful). Our work, then, while bearing witness to the importance, usefulness and practical applicability of arts and humanities research in crisis contexts, also situates itself within broader national and international debates about the role arts and humanities play in fostering and sustaining the creative and open-ended critical thinking that underpins democratic political structures.

The *Pandemic and Beyond* series

The aim of this series is to preserve the breadth of the approaches taken by *Pandemic and Beyond* researchers in addressing the crisis, showcasing a form of arts and humanities research that has learned how to respond to, and mitigate, COVID-19 as it unfolded, and that has constantly adapted its methods and research questions to ongoing developments and the needs of research participants. Reflecting the variety of the *Pandemic and Beyond* research portfolio, the chapters we have selected range from in-depth reflection on schools of thought and social and governance structures that have influenced approaches to the pandemic to those that are much more 'hands-on'. These latter chapters address subjects sometimes sidelined in conventional academic writing, as their focus on working structures, industrial practices and lived experience does not always lend itself easily to conceptual debates and theorisation.

Written from the retrospective vantage point of late 2022 and the first months of 2023, these chapters offer a rare insight into the findings and often invisible facets of research projects whose primary focus was rapid on-the-ground impact, knowledge exchange, and direct engagement with communities, organisations and decision-makers. The chapters we collect not only offer reflection on what the research teams achieved, but also on what could be learned from their experiences to guide future responses to ongoing, accelerating and emerging crises, whether in relation to climate, migration, violent conflict, the threat of vaccine-resistant coronavirus variants, or other pathogens that could develop into new pandemics. The result is a series which models how, in responding to a crisis, the creativity, cultural sensitivity, community-reach and knowledge base of arts and humanities researchers can be one of the best tools to understand a novel virus in all its dimensions, steer policy and alleviate suffering on the ground.

In our volume *Adaptation and Resilience in the Performing Arts*, we explore how live performing arts in the UK innovated during public health restrictions to everyday life to overcome the obstacles to co-presence and performance in shared spaces that were a side-effect of pandemic mitigation measures. The volume explores the financial hardship and mental health impacts experienced by industry professionals as governmental discourses regarding the 'viability' of arts careers, alongside the difficulties of connecting with networks and accessing arts opportunities, put a particular strain on creative workers and freelancers in the UK at a time when some Latin American countries were leading the way in valuing and supporting the arts. Against this backdrop of existential struggle for creative workers, this volume celebrates the ingenuity and creativity of artists and researchers who applied themselves to finding both digital and analogue solutions to the problem of co-presence, and who, in so doing, broadened the access of previously marginalised communities to live performing arts. It highlights projects that explored how motion-capture and green screen technologies can enable performers to come together despite geographical distance and interact in a shared virtual space to create new work, and how such digital work affects their art, wellbeing and ability to reach wider audiences. It also champions the value of local initiatives in outdoor spaces and suggests avenues for artists and local governments to reimagine towns and cities as performance venues in which diverse communities can gather to celebrate their location and ability to communally enjoy art amid a pandemic.

The mobilisation of existing natural, community and cultural assets and resources to support individual and community wellbeing – conducted at speed and often using novel modes of delivery – was a notable feature of pandemic responses across the UK. Our volume *Creative Approaches to Wellbeing* presents detailed examples of research looking at how these kinds of activities sought to address issues such as the challenges of isolation, to support health and care workers, or to create spaces that could enable coping, recovery or renewal. Common to the chapters here are reflections on what it means and what tools and systems might be needed if we are to develop resilience during and after such crises in future, alongside examination of ideas of 'vulnerability'. Authors bring to these discussions a particular focus on the experiences of those most marginalised during the pandemic because of mental or physical ill-health, age, or due to deep-seated structural and systemic inequalities. Individual contributions include an interrogation of the idea of 'togetherness' itself; an invitation to consider the benefits of 'walking creatively', a study of the work of small organisations in promoting health through interaction with urban nature; and investigations of the contributions of the cultural, museum and literary heritage sectors to wellbeing. Looking forward, authors invite us to consider how adaptations to ways of working for individuals, within organisations, and even at the level of a whole city region, could lead to changes in provision and lessons for practice.

Knowing COVID-19 looks at how different kinds of knowledge and meaning have been created and communicated, and the repercussions this has had – and continues to have – for how COVID-19 is managed, experienced, understood and remembered. Knowledge-making, it suggests, took various forms, and these are reflected in the diversity of chapters this volume curates. In the first instance, it demonstrates a rich humanities tradition of constructive critique, as 'official' communications around 'staying home', 'keeping distance', safety on buses, lateral flow testing, and vaccine hesitancy are tested and interrogated. Through this collective work, we see one of the clear, indisputable values of the humanities; their attentiveness to the human, and the clarifying or reflective power this might have had with greater embeddedness in policy and information design. In the second instance – and frequently both are accomplished in the same short chapter – this volume collects a series of interventions which set out specifically to create and sustain meaning, particularly when dominant cultural narratives over the pandemic rely on those meanings slipping away from political or popular memory. Thus, we have rich and detailed explorations of the experiences of museum workers, people told to 'stay home', older victims of gender-based violence, people with deafblindness, and racialised nurses working in the NHS; as well as extensive reflection on what it was like to make the projects which formalised this knowledge work. Taken as a whole, this volume critiques and redefines pandemic epistemologies, assembling a partial blueprint for making future crises legible.

Finally, *Governance, Democracy and Ethics in Crisis-Decision-Making* explores what it means to be in a situation in which rational or epistemic framings of the COVID-19 pandemic, with a focus on data and scientific ways of knowing the world, rub up against more entangled accounts. In these accounts, humans, the virus and governance arrangements coexist as a broader, relational whole. Human connections, personal fulfilment and social groupings are inextricably intertwined with matters (and meanings) of governance, ethics and authority, the rule of law, the economy and, crucially, public health. Looking at issues ranging from the authority of the WHO and the power of data during an emergency, to the role of public engagement as a source of policy evidence, we reflect on what it means to govern *ethically* in a pandemic, and whether the expected standards and norms of public life, evidence and decision-making should be different in times of crisis. We also reflect on how the long tail of the pandemic seems impossible to disentangle from a reduced trust in power and authority, creating an urgent need for ethics to move beyond normative assertions of the law and regulations. Our authors provide some suggestions as to how these things might be balanced more ethically and effectively in the future.

In 2020 and 2021, when televised government briefings on COVID-19 remained commonplace, ministers insisted time and again that they were 'following the science' (Colman et al., 2021). Even when critics called the accuracy of this rhetorical device into question, they rarely troubled the governing logic that, were we only willing to follow it, scientific and medical evidence offered an unclouded route map through the pandemic. However, '[c]oping with the pandemic was (for the lucky majority who were not severely ill) not so much a medical crisis as an existential one' (Thain et al., 2023: 13); indeed, given the complex interplay of social, cultural, ethical, economic and political framings of health, illness and disease, there is no such thing as a purely medical crisis (Ryan, 2022). The *Pandemic and Beyond* series reveals how the arts and humanities research community rose to the challenge of this complexity, growing in confidence as it became increasingly clear that our methodologies, forms of knowledge and creative mindsets were key not only to tackling this all-encompassing human emergency, but, in so doing, to alleviating human suffering. As one of our researchers commented:

> What has been evident across our COVID-19 research projects is that arts-based research methods and approaches can generate much more nuanced narratives, capture the complex experiences and engage people that wouldn't otherwise find research accessible. Whilst of course medical research in such a crisis is fundamental, so too is understanding different people's experiences, responses and how their lives have been impacted so we can make more effective policies and support people's recovery and resilience looking forward. (Aebischer et al., 2022: 30)

If, as another *Pandemic and Beyond* researcher put it, this work 'has been a game-changer' in revealing the skill and generosity of the research community (Aebischer et al., 2022: 29), then it is also a call to action in the future, as we face a multitude of ongoing and emerging crises, from climate to migration and economic decline, which demand collective and civic responsibility and the willingness to continue to combine nuanced and context-sensitive thinking with a solutions-focused approach.

Without the vast collective knowledge, experience, methodological tools and expertise on which this type of research draws, our responses to ongoing challenges and future crises can only ever be impoverished. Expecting politicians of the future to say that they are 'following the humanities' might be wishful thinking. A pandemic response which made more extensive use of the kinds of evidence and interventions on show in these volumes, however, would have been far more attentive to questions of power and justice; understood how, why and when particular people felt – and became – less safe; had a far better handle on how we engage with public health advice or vaccination drives; and begun from a richer knowledge of what the arts can do to keep us feeling human in the most difficult of circumstances. As a recent essay on climate change suggests, the arts and humanities have to be equal to the series of interlocking emergencies which frame our present historical moment (Pietsch and Flanagan, 2020). Over the past three years, scholars and practitioners have painstakingly built a 'pandemic humanities' – and a pandemic arts and cultural sector – which demonstrates that the arts and humanities are more than equal to the task. Creating the conditions for this work to (continue to) thrive must, surely, constitute one of the best forms of crisis preparedness we have.

Notes

1 Funded by UKRI/AHRC from February 2021 to February 2022, grant reference AH/W000881/1. The project's legacy website is housed at https://pandemicandbeyond.exeter.ac.uk/ and will be maintained until February 2028.
2 *The Pandemic and Beyond* was responsible specifically for the AHRC segment of the research portfolio created by the UKRI call, first published on 31 March 2020, for 'ideas that address COVID-19'. A version of the call updated on 21 September 2020 is available at www.ukri.org/opportunity/get-funding-for-ideas-that-address-covid-19/ (last accessed 4 February 2023).
3 For a map of projects focusing on COVID-19 funded by UKRI, see https://strategicfutures.org/TopicMaps/UKRI/research_map.html (last accessed 4 February 2023).

References

Aebischer, P. et al. (2022) 'The pandemic and beyond: the arts and humanities contribution to covid research and recovery', Final Project Report. Available at: http://hdl.handle.net/10871/132640 (accessed 30 March 2023).

Baraitser, L. and Salisbury, L. (2020) '"Containment, delay, mitigation": waiting and care in the time of a pandemic' [version 2; peer review: 2 approved], *Wellcome Open Research*, 5: 129. https://doi.org/10.12688/wellcomeopenres.15970.2

Callard, F. and Perego, E. (2021) 'How and why patients made Long Covid', *Social Science and Medicine*, 268: 113426. https://doi.org/10.1016/j.socscimed.2020.113426

Colman, E. et al. (2021) 'Following the science? Views from scientists on government advisory boards during the COVID-19 pandemic: a qualitative interview study in five European Countries', *BMJ Global Health*, 6: e006928. https://doi.org/10.1136/bmjgh-2021-006928

Fowler, D. (2020) 'Unemployment during coronavirus: the psychology of job loss', *BBC Worklife*, 28 March. Available at: www.bbc.com/worklife/article/20200327-unemployment-during-coronavirus-the-psychology-of-job-loss (accessed 30 February 2023).

Greene, J. A. and Vargha, D. (2020) 'How epidemics end', *Boston Review*, 30 June 2020. Available at: www.bostonreview.net/articles/jeremy-greene-dora-vargha-how-epidemics-end-or-dont/ (accessed 30 March 2023).

Gupta, S., Rouse, B. T. and Sarangi, P. P. (2021) 'Did climate change influence the emergence, transmission, and expression of the COVID-19 pandemic?', *Frontiers in Medicine*, 8: 769208. https://doi.org/10.3389/fmed.2021.769208

King, J. and Ferraz, O. (eds) (2021–23) *The Oxford Compendium of National Legal Responses to COVID-19*, Oxford Constitutional Law. Available at: https://oxcon.ouplaw.com/home/OCC19 (accessed 4 February 2023).

Pietsch, T. and Flanagan, F. (2020) 'Here we stand: temporal thinking in urgent times', *History Australia*, 17(2): 252–271. https://doi.org/10.1080/14490854.2020.1758577

Pirgova-Morgan, L. (2022) 'Exploring the impact of COVID-19 on GCRF and Newton Projects: a research report by PRAXIS: Arts and Humanities for Global Development', University of Leeds: PRAXIS: Arts and Humanities for Global Development. Available at: https://changingthestory.leeds.ac.uk/wp-content/uploads/sites/178/2022/06/University-of-Leeds-PRAXIS-COVID-19-Report-Final-Single-0422.pdf (accessed 30 March 2023).

Qureshi, I. et al. (2022) 'Healthcare workers from diverse ethnicities and their perceptions of risk and experiences of risk management during the COVID-19 pandemic: qualitative insights from the United Kingdom-REACH study', *Frontiers in Medicine*, 9: 930904. https://doi.org/10.3389/fmed.2022.930904

Ryan, J. Michael (2022) 'Coda: global consciousness of COVID-19: where can we go from here?', in I. Gammel and J. Wang (eds) *Creative Resilience and COVID-19: Figuring the Everyday in a Pandemic*, Abingdon: Routledge, 195–200.

Shakespeare, T., Ndagire, F. and Seketi, Q. E. (2021) 'Triple jeopardy: disabled people and the COVID-19 pandemic', *The Lancet* 397(10282): 1331–1333. https://doi.org/10.1016/S0140-6736(21)00625-5

Thain, M. et al. (2023) 'The humanities in the UK today: what's going on?', *HEPI Report* 159, March. Available at: www.hepi.ac.uk/wp-content/uploads/2023/03/The-Humanities-in-the-UK-Today-Whats-Going-On.pdf (accessed 30 March 2023).

WEF (2021) 'Covid employment global job loss', World Economic Forum, 4 February. Available at: www.weforum.org/agenda/2021/02/covid-employment-global-job-loss/ (accessed 20 February 2023).

WHO (2022a) 'COVID-19 pandemic triggers 25% increase in prevalence of anxiety and depression worldwide', WHO News Release, 2 March. Available at: www.who.int/news/item/02-03-2022-covid-19-pandemic-triggers-25-increase-in-prevalence-of-anxiety-and-depression-worldwide (accessed 20 February 2023).

WHO (2022b) 'Two million confirmed deaths from COVID-19 in the European region', WHO News Release, 12 May. Available at: www.who.int/europe/news/item/12-05-2022-two-million-confirmed-deaths-from-covid-19-in-the-european-region (accessed 20 February 2023).

Figures and tables

Figure

6.1 Arnstein's Ladder of Citizen Participation   128

Tables

2.1 Relationships and ethical values in healthcare decision-making   48
7.1 Seven principles for successful public health emergency decision-making and governance   165

Contributors

Pascale Aebischer, Professor of Shakespeare and Early Modern Performance Studies, University of Exeter. *The Pandemic and Beyond: The Arts and Humanities Contribution to COVID Research and Recovery* (AH/W000881/1); *Digital Theatre Transformation: A Case Study and Digital Toolkit for Small to Mid-Scale Companies in England* (AH/V008102/1).

Rachel Allsopp, Assistant Professor, Northumbria Law School, Northumbria University Newcastle. *The Observatory for Monitoring Data-Driven Approaches to COVID-19 (OMDDAC)* (AH/V012789/1).

Claire Bessant, Associate Professor, Northumbria Law School, Northumbria University Newcastle. *The Observatory for Monitoring Data-Driven Approaches to COVID-19 (OMDDAC)* (AH/V012789/1).

Anna Chiumento, Lecturer in Global Mental Health and Society, The University of Edinburgh. *When pandemic and everyday ethics collide: supporting ethical decision-making in maternity care and paediatrics during the Covid-19 pandemic* (AH/V00820X/1).

Fred Cooper, Senior Research Associate for Epistemic Injustice in Health Care Project (EPIC), University of Bristol. *Scenes of Shame and Stigma in COVID-19* (AH/V013483/1).

Heather Draper, Professor of Bioethics, Warwick Medical School, University of Warwick. *When pandemic and everyday ethics* *collide: supporting ethical decision-making in maternity care and paediatrics during the Covid-19 pandemic* (AH/V00820X/1).

Mark Eccleston-Turner, Senior Lecturer in Global Health Law, King's College, London. *Assessing the viability of access and benefit-sharing models of equitable distribution of vaccines in international law* (AH/V006924/1).

Des Fitzgerald, Professor of Medical Humanities and Social Sciences, Radical Humanities Laboratory, University College Cork. *The Pandemic and Beyond: The Arts and Humanities Contribution to COVID Research and Recovery* (AH/W000881/1).

Sara Fovargue, Professor of Law, the University of Sheffield. *When pandemic and everyday ethics collide: supporting ethical decision-making in maternity care and paediatrics during the Covid-19 pandemic* (AH/V00820X/1).

Lucy Frith, Reader in Bioethics, Centre for Social Ethics and Policy, The University of Manchester. *When pandemic and everyday ethics collide: supporting ethical decision-making in maternity care and paediatrics during the Covid-19 pandemic* (AH/V00820X/1).

Karen Gray, Senior Research Associate, School of Policy Studies, University of Bristol. *COVID-19: Impacts on the Cultural Industries and Implications for Policy* (AH/V00994X/1); *The Pandemic and Beyond: The Arts and Humanities Contribution to COVID Research and Recovery* (AH/W000881/1).

Abbie-Rose Hampton, PhD student, Department of Global Health & Social Medicine, King's College London. *Assessing the viability of access and benefit-sharing models of equitable distribution of vaccines in international law* (AH/V006924/1).

Daniel Herron, Head of Research Innovation at University College London Hospital. *UK Pandemic Ethics Accelerator* (AH/V013947/1).

Jack Hume, PhD student, Department of Philosophy, University College, London. *UK Pandemic Ethics Accelerator* (AH/V013947/1).

Kiran Kaur Manku, DPhil student, NDM Centre for Global Health Research, University of Oxford. *UK Pandemic Ethics Accelerator* (AH/V013947/1).

Lina Minou, Research Fellow, Department of Philosophy, University College, London. *UK Pandemic Ethics Accelerator* (AH/V013947/1).

Cian O'Donovan, Senior Research Fellow, Department of Science and Technology Studies, University College London. *UK Pandemic Ethics Accelerator* (AH/V013947/1).

Reema Patel, Research Director and Head of Deliberative Engagement at Ipsos UK. *The role of good governance and the rule of law in building public trust in data-driven responses to public health emergencies* (AH/V015214/1).

Caroline Redhead, Research Fellow, Centre for Social Ethics and Policy, The University of Manchester. *When pandemic and everyday ethics collide: supporting ethical decision-making in maternity care and paediatrics during the Covid-19 pandemic* (AH/V00820X/1).

Melanie Smallman, Associate Professor, Department of Science & Technology Studies, University College London. *UK Pandemic Ethics Accelerator* (AH/V013947/1).

Victoria Tischler, Professor of Behavioural Science, Faculty of Health and Medical Sciences, University of Surrey. *Using Multisensory Culture Boxes to Promote Public Health Guidance and to Support the Wellbeing of People with Dementia in Care Homes* (AH/V006991/2); *The Pandemic and Beyond: The Arts and Humanities Contribution to COVID Research and Recovery* (AH/W000881/1).

Harry Upton, PhD student, Department of Global Health & Social Medicine, King's College London. *Assessing the viability of access and benefit-sharing models of equitable distribution of vaccines in international law* (AH/V006924/1).

Jamie Webb, PhD student, Centre for Technomoral Futures, the University of Edinburgh. *UK Pandemic Ethics Accelerator* (AH/V013947/1).

James Wilson, Professor of Philosophy, University College London. *UK Pandemic Ethics Accelerator* (AH/V013947/1).

Acknowledgements

The editors would like to thank the Arts and Humanities Research Council for funding *The Pandemic and Beyond*. We extend our thanks to Pascale Aebischer for her wisdom and energetic support throughout our shaping of this book and, indeed, *The Pandemic and Beyond* series as a whole. We would also like to recognise the contribution of Sarah Hartley, who was Caroline's original co-editor.

We would both like to thank our colleagues – from the Reset Ethics research project (Caroline) and the Pandemic Ethics Accelerator team (Melanie) – for support and encouragement with the work of bringing this book to fruition, as well as their more tangible contributions to its contents.

Introduction

Melanie Smallman and Caroline Redhead

The sight of the British Prime Minister lining up with his scientific and medical advisers in the Downing Street briefing room became very familiar to UK citizens during the early stages of the coronavirus (COVID-19) pandemic – the time that the research brought together in *The Pandemic and Beyond* was being carried out. Each day, three men shared a series of graphs and diagrams to explain the progress and development of the disease, the Prime Minister even going as far as to claim to be guided by 'Data not dates' (BBC News, 2021). The pandemic was being seen very much as an epistemic and technical problem. What do we know about this new virus, to what level of certainty, and how does that guide us to act – or not to act? In the Introduction to Volume 1 in this series, *Knowing COVID-19: The Pandemic and Beyond*, Fred Cooper and Des Fitzgerald noted that, in being 'guided by the science' (GOV. UK, 2020), zooming in on 'data not dates', COVID-19 decision-makers de-prioritised the importance of *human* stories about meaning and experience. In the pandemic world, the world of the briefing room, of the graphs and diagrams, people and viruses alike comprised the data points to be studied, counted, governed and regulated, individual pieces to be reorganised according to algorithmic and scientific outputs. The focus in Volume 1 was on how humanities expertise can be a part of producing new knowledge on a novel infectious disease. In Volume 4, our focus is on how humanities research can inform and support better decision-making in the next pandemic.

Having started inside the briefing room, we now look outside. We zoom out from the graphs and diagrams, expanding the focus from the data points to the *people* they represent. This is the world in which the humanities researchers, whose contributions shape this book, were bringing their expertise to bear. The conversations we had with our research participants were often difficult, and occasionally emotional, as we worked together to understand what was going on. New or developing research methods were sometimes employed as researchers worked to bridge the gap between descriptions of what *was* happening and what people thought *ought to be* happening (see, for example, Frith, 2012). People outside the briefing room were living and working in a very different pandemic world; a messier and more entangled world. In this world, people's stories co-existed with stories about the virus, about the suffering and sacrifices of 'key workers', and about people dying alone. In no sense was co-existence with the virus an individual affair. Instead, people were intra-acting as components of communities that pulled together wherever they could, supporting each other, virtually where that was all that was permitted, and forming a broader, relational whole that was much larger than the sum of the parts.

But as infection rates climbed, human connections, personal fulfilment, social groupings and leisure activities inexorably became intertwined with matters of governance and authority, the rule (and role) of law and legality, the economy and the markets, as well as public health, infection prevention measures – and the virus itself. Questions of ethics moved far beyond well-trodden normative assertions of rights and wrongs, upheld by predictable and transparent laws and regulatory processes. In this world of uncertainty, fear of infection and death loomed large. Where authoritarian lockdowns prevented social interaction, with the size of permitted gatherings seeming to reduce on a weekly basis, people understood the necessity for draconian measures and (generally) complied. After all, we were all in this together, weren't we?

That, in fact, we weren't all in it together was soon to become clear. The revelation that Boris Johnson, the (then) Prime Minister had hosted numerous gatherings in his home and office while the rest of the country had been in lockdown raised questions about his moral credibility, and the general fitness of many of his ministerial colleagues to occupy public office. In their recent book, Fred Cooper and colleagues (2023) describe how a patterning of shame and shaming emerged within the UK's pandemic landscape. They discuss, through a series of case studies, how experiences of shame, shaming and stigma dominated personal and public life during the COVID-19 pandemic, with the use of terms like 'COVIDiot' seeing people divided into categories of morally worthy or morally unworthy, and being shamed or praised accordingly. Importantly, rather than minimising this, they argue that the UK government's actions actually worsened this trend. Offering a 'COVID-19 and shame timeline 2020' (Cooper et al., 2023: vii–xii), they situate the 'shameful' personal actions of the Prime Minister and other senior public figures within the broader catalogue of rules and restrictions imposed on everyone else, asking why public officials felt it necessary to deflect shame from themselves regardless of the public health consequences.

Elsewhere in the growing corpus of COVID-19 literature, to which this book contributes, academics are examining the many aspects and implications of pandemic decision-making across various aspects of life, society and democracy. Emphasising the inter- and intra-connectedness of virus, people and place, we find, for example, literature discussing microbiology and the built environment and how the decision-making of both public officials and homeowners might change following the pandemic (Dietz et al., 2020). Academic commentary suggests that, in looking to the future more broadly, experiences of the pandemic have changed the notion of 'community' (Alberti, 2020), and that people want different things from their leaders now (Youngs, 2020). Suggesting that democracy is the missing link in European Union recovery plans, Youngs advocates for stronger democratic participation as a positive and helpful part of the post-virus rebuilding phase. Similarly, Parry et al. (2020) describe how democratic spaces were reconfigured during COVID-19, noting how participatory spaces shrank, overlapped and invaded each other and concluding that democracies are generally not prepared to sustain deliberation and participation in times of crisis. For this reason, participation needs to be further institutionalised. Many contributors to this book, drawing on their investigations of pandemic decision-making, echo this call.

Alongside an examination of pandemic governance in academic literature and commentary, the decision-making behind pandemic rules and restrictions in the UK is, at the time of writing, subject to review by various official bodies, including the UK COVID-19

Inquiry and the Independent Commission on UK Public Health Emergency Powers.[1] Emphasising the need for a detailed reflection on decision-making during the pandemic, the House of Lords Select Committee on the Constitution (Constitution Committee) had noted, in June 2021 that, while exceptional measures had been necessary to limit the spread of COVID-19 and keep communities safe, many of the decisions that had transformed everyday life by imposing unprecedented restrictions on ordinary activities had been made with extremely limited parliamentary oversight (House of Lords, 2021). As a result, the Constitution Committee recommended that a review of the use of emergency powers by the government, and the (lack of) scrutiny of those powers by parliament, should be undertaken. The Constitution Committee was particularly keen to emphasise that the approach adopted in response to the pandemic *must not* be used to justify weakened parliamentary scrutiny of government action in response to any future emergencies (House of Lords, 2021; emphasis added). In response to the Constitution Committee's report, the Independent Commission on UK Public Health Emergency Powers (the Emergency Powers Commission) was convened. The Emergency Powers Commission has a broad remit to provide a legal and constitutional analysis of existing and alternative emergency public health laws, parliamentary procedures for responding to public health emergencies, and the ways in which emergency laws and public health guidance were made, scrutinised, utilised and disseminated during the COVID-19 pandemic (British Institute of International and Comparative Law, 2023).[2]

The work of the Emergency Powers Commission bridges the briefing room world and the messier human world in some respects. Among the issues it will examine are, for instance, the extent to which government messaging distinguished between *binding law* and *non-binding public health advice*. This subtle distinction appeared to be blurred further by those implicated in the Partygate events, as they sought to avoid any accusations of wrongdoing (UK Parliament, 2023) but also stimulated discussion outside the briefing room about exceptional executive powers in an emergency, the role of trust, and the importance of the principles of good governance – such as selflessness, integrity, accountability and honesty in leadership.

In this book we explore these issues further. Specifically, we consider what it means to be in a decision-making situation whereby rational or epistemic framings of the COVID-19 pandemic, with a focus on data and scientific ways of knowing the world, rub up against more entangled human experiences and existences. How can (or should) we re-focus our perspectives and our systems as a result? Looking at matters ranging from the authority of the World Health Organization (WHO) and the power of data during an emergency, to the role of public engagement as a source of policy evidence, we reflect on what it means to govern ethically in a pandemic, and whether (and how) the expected standards and norms of public life, evidence and decision-making apply in such circumstances. We also reflect on how power, authority, trust and the sense of the ending of the pandemic are inextricably linked, creating a need for ethics to move beyond normative assertions of the law and regulations, whether in hospitals or in the halls of parliamentary power.

Bringing together findings from *The Pandemic and Beyond* research projects (all of which were carried out while the pandemic was unfolding), the chapters that follow reflect the voices of the authors' research participants as they consider how we can grapple, collectively, with such challenges. All of the chapters are linked by a focus on how decisions have been made, but nevertheless look at the pandemic from very different perspectives. In this way, we produce a series of different portraits of pandemic decision-making that are marbled through with various common themes relating to ethics, values, governance, trust and inclusion. Indeed, some of these themes can be traced through the entire series. For instance, in their introduction to *Adaptation and Resilience in the Performing Arts: The Pandemic and Beyond*, Pascale Aebischer and Rachael Nicholas highlight values of inclusion, community, innovation, equity and care that inform their authors' reflections on the impacts of the pandemic. Similar guiding reflections underpin the chapters that follow in this book, as our authors explore decision-making processes ranging from the everyday to the global.

More specifically, the chapters draw out discussions relating to the importance of values and ethics, both of which take on extra importance in the context of public health decision-making, where decisions can have *physical* impacts on human bodies. The importance of institutional structures of governance and scrutiny – and the consequences of their neglect – are thrown into sharp relief, as is the crucial importance of involving diverse voices in decision-making, acknowledging that the effects of the pandemic are not felt in the same way by different individuals, groups or communities. Collectively, the chapters reveal wider sociological lessons about how social and institutional arrangements (along with the virus itself) have co-produced (and undermined) power and authority, and how this has amplified some voices while sidelining or even silencing others. This book thus highlights the crucial role of humanities research in helping us look beyond 'the science', exposing and exploring the plural pathways that link microbial organisms and humans; children and data; decision-making and infection prevention. We consider how the pandemic could have been otherwise and offer a series of perspectives on how, now and into the future, governance, democracy and ethics in crisis-decision-making must change.

The book starts with a chapter by Lina Minou, James Wilson and Daniel Herron, who question how we understand the 'form' of an epidemic (and by extension, a pandemic). Reflecting on the relationship between the intellectual constructs of the epidemic phenomenon and its meaning as an occurrence within an individual life, they argue that while a key feature of an epidemic is the way in which cases of infection suddenly arise and then fall, in reality pinpointing these precise points is difficult and anyway does not do justice to the meaning of an epidemic for an individual as a life-event. Instead, they argue that the complexity of the several manifestations of the epidemic reality demands an equally complex conceptual framework. In a *pandemic*, understood as a collection of interconnected epidemics, or an epidemic that travels, this complexity is amplified. In warning against the danger of presenting too linear and too homogeneous an understanding of pandemics, the authors set the scene in Chapter 1 for the chapters that follow, which tell the different stories of governance and decision-making that have emerged from the research projects represented in the volume.

Chapter 2 starts with tales from the fight against COVID-19 in National Health Service (NHS) hospitals in the UK. Caroline Redhead, Anna Chiumento, Sara Fovargue, Heather Draper and Lucy Frith explore the everyday ethical challenges faced by staff as NHS maternity and paediatrics services were 'reset' during the pandemic. Such challenges were often embedded in changes to working practices intended to keep staff safe, and to protect hospital communities from COVID-19 infection. However, these changes reduced healthcare professionals' ability to 'care' for their patients, where care is understood as embracing the interpersonal relationships between the patient (and their family) and the healthcare team. Although they protected healthcare staff and patients from COVID-19, infection prevention and control measures caused harm by creating barriers to relational interaction and engagement. In this chapter, the authors consider the significance of relationships in a healthcare context. They describe the theoretical underpinnings of a logic of *relationality* in healthcare, which they argue should underpin healthcare decision-making.

In Chapter 3, the focus shifts from healthcare to social care. Rather than providing care in the context of treatment for a medical condition, social care is about offering people support with their day-to-day needs, whether they arise from illness, disability, old age or poverty. In the UK, the social care 'system' distributes responsibilities and obligations for this type of support between the welfare state, voluntary sectors and communities, and families. In this chapter, Cian O'Donovan describes and discusses the significant existing problems in social care data infrastructures, and how these were exacerbated and amplified by government decision-making during the pandemic. Starting from the catastrophic government decision to discharge people from hospitals into care homes for the elderly without considering the significant risks of COVID-19 transmission, the author considers how social care data systems could better support outcomes for care home residents and social care requirements more generally.

Data use during the pandemic is also the focus of Chapter 4, in which Melanie Smallman, Cian O'Donovan, James Wilson and Jack Hume ask whether data ethics have been a casualty of the pandemic. Describing three key 'episodes' in the COVID-19 pandemic where data played a key role – and which raised significant ethical issues – they demonstrate how emergency measures were intimately linked with the collection and analysis of data at an accelerated pace, and how data formed a key part of the logic by which power was wielded over the public. They argue that the authority given by the seeming objectivity of data was sufficiently powerful to enable the British Prime Minister and government to enact, and then repeal (arguably too quickly), severe restrictions on civil liberties in the UK, in some instances appearing to bypass the relevant ethical advisory boards and escape the scrutiny of 'traditional' data ethics frameworks. Drawing parallels to the regulation of drugs research during a pandemic, they conclude that a set of 'emergency data ethics' is needed to help guide thinking in a future such emergency.

In Chapter 5, the centrality of data-driven decision-making to the UK government's response to COVID-19 is considered from the perspective of children. Claire Bessant and Rachel Allsopp, working with child rights organisation, Investing in Children, as part of the Observatory for Monitoring Data-Driven Approaches to COVID-19, describe young people's views about how their data was used during the pandemic. They note that government decisions (to close schools, to introduce lockdowns, social distancing and self-isolation requirements, and to determine exam results using flawed algorithms) have had a significant impact upon children and young people's mental and physical health and wellbeing and upon their education, negatively affecting children's rights. Reporting that more work is clearly needed to ensure that young people's views are heard and their stories told, this chapter incorporates the voices of young people into the authors' recommendations to policymakers for engaging effectively with this vital section of the population.

Continuing the theme of missing voices in government decision-making, the focus of Chapter 6 is on pandemic public policy-making in the UK. Lamenting the absence of the public voice in ethically laden policy choices, such as vaccine prioritisation, Jamie Webb and Kiran Kaur Manku consider how the 'public' has been characterised in, how publics were present or absent from, and whether publics were consulted as part of decision-making during the COVID-19 crisis. By interrogating the theoretical underpinnings and ethical justifications for practical engagement with publics, the authors suggest avenues for more proactive public engagement in the continuing COVID-19 response as well as in planning for the pandemics to come.

In Chapter 7, Reema Patel widens the focus on the theme of missing voices in government to a global perspective. She notes that the onset of COVID-19 resulted in the majority of democratic nation states worldwide implementing a state of emergency, often without widespread societal debate or discussion in key democratic spaces such as parliamentary chambers. Thus, democratic public participation in national decision-making was a casualty elsewhere as well as in the UK. The author contends that this created contradictory messaging – on the one hand, appealing to the core concepts of democracy and the rule of law to ask for public compliance and support, but on the other, actively undermining these core concepts by overstepping their legal authority in various ways. She suggests that the result was a crisis of confidence in the pandemic response, rather than confidence in a crisis. Drawing from a wide range of examples and the deliberations of two UK citizen juries considering the fundamentals of good governance, she argues that in future crises, democratic nation states need to create participatory infrastructures for democracy in a crisis to complement (and act as a check on) the risks of executive power overreach through the blunt instrument of emergency decision-making.

Continuing the global perspective, Chapter 8 considers the use of emergency powers by the WHO, exploring the extent to which the use of these powers aligns with principles of good global health governance. Harry Upton, Abbie-Rose Hampton and Mark Eccleston-Turner outline why good governance matters for international organisations, suggesting that, while the COVID-19 pandemic has emphasised the vital importance of an effective and efficient coordinated response to emerging health threats on a global scale, it has also demonstrated that the current system ultimately lacks the means and mechanisms through which to ensure good global health governance within and between key organisations in global health, most notably the WHO itself.

To conclude, an important point we want to leave readers of this volume to ponder is the question of whether or not we need special measures for making decisions in a pandemic (or similar such emergency). A number of the chapters in this volume flag up insufficiencies in the way in which decisions were made during the early stages of the COVID-19 pandemic in the UK. For instance, in Chapter 5, Claire Bessant and Rachel Allsopp argue that data-driven decision-making produced policies that disproportionately harmed children and young people, without offering them a voice in return. The authors advocate for better engagement with young people in future. Similarly, in Chapters 6 and 7, Jamie Webb, Kiran Kaur Manku and Reema Patel argue that increased public engagement in decision-making would have helped make better decisions – not least by strengthening the voices of those overlooked and perhaps worst affected by the pandemic. But what remains unclear is whether these insufficiencies were the result of the *absence* of mechanisms by which these voices or perspectives *could* have been brought into consideration, whether they were simply inappropriate under such urgent and straightened conditions, or, as Melanie Smallman, Cian O'Donovan, James Wilson and Jack Hume argue in Chapter 4 was the case with ethics advice, the checks and balances that *were* in place to ensure good policymaking were neglected, ignored or overridden by political leaders in this instance. In other words, was the pandemic the extraordinary condition from which we learn systemic lessons, or, rather, did the tone set by the government of the day marginalise, disable or ignore systems and processes that were already sufficiently dynamic and flexible to have enabled a different approach?

Perhaps history (together with the outcome of the UK COVID-19 Inquiry and the work of the Public Health Commission, both ongoing at the time of writing) will enable us to make a better judgement on this. Suffice, for now, to say that gaining a clearer picture of the extent to which the COVID-19 pandemic in the UK was an 'ordinary emergency' (as Lina Minou, James Wilson and Daniel Herron put it in their chapter) or whether there were other factors at play significant in creating an *extra*ordinary situation (such as might be argued to have been the case for the healthcare professionals whose experiences informed the discussion in Chapter 2). The answers to these questions will be vital in understanding how we all need to reflect upon our pandemic life-event experiences of the last few years. Maybe, as we emerge from the pandemic through, and as a result of, accepting our entangled intra-relationships, the lessons drawn out in this volume will support decision-makers in both ordinary times and extraordinary emergencies.

Notes

1 See https://covid19.public-inquiry.uk/ and https://binghamcentre.biicl. org/independent-commission-on-uk-public-health-emergency-powers, respectively.
2 Reema Patel, the author of Chapter 7, sits as one of the Commissioners on the Public Health Commission: https://binghamcentre.biicl.org/meet-the-commissioner-uk-public-health-emergency-powers

References

Alberti, F. (2020) 'Coronavirus is revitalising the concept of community for the 21st century', *The Conversation*. Available at: https://theconversation.com/coronavirus-is-revitalising-the-concept-of-community-for-the-21st-century-135750 (accessed 19 May 2023).

BBC News (2021) 'Covid: Boris Johnson to focus on "data, not dates" for lockdown easing', *BBC News*, 17 February. Available at: www.bbc.com/news/uk-56095552 (accessed 11 May 2023).

British Institute of International and Comparative Law (2023) 'Independent Commission on UK Public Health Emergency Powers'. Available at: https://binghamcentre.biicl.org/independent-commission-on-uk-public-health-emergency-powers (accessed 11 May 2023).

Cooper, F., Dolezal, L. and Rose, A. (2023) *COVID-19 and Shame: Political Emotions and Public Health in the UK* (Critical Interventions in the Medical and Health Humanities), London: Bloomsbury Academic. Available at: http://dx.doi.org.manchester.idm.oclc.org/10.5040/9781350283442 (accessed 11 May 2023).

Dietz, L. et al. (2020) '2019 novel coronavirus (COVID-19) pandemic: built environment considerations to reduce transmission', *mSystems*, 5(2). Available at: https://doi.org/10.1128/mSystems.00245-20 (accessed 19 May 2023).

Frith, L. (2012) 'Symbiotic empirical ethics: a practical methodology', *Bioethics*, 26(4): 190–206.

GOV.UK (2020) 'Prime Minister's statement on coronavirus (COVID-19)', 18 March. Available at: www.gov.uk/government/speeches/pm-statement-on-coronavirus-18-march-2020 (accessed 11 May 2023).

House of Lords (2021) 'COVID-19 and the use and scrutiny of emergency powers', Select Committee on the Constitution 3rd Report of Session 2021–22: HL Paper 15. Available at: https://committees.parliament.uk/publications/6212/documents/69015/default/ (accessed 11 May 2023).

Parry, L. J., Asenbaum, H. and Ercan, S. A. (2020) 'Democracy in flux: a systemic view on the impact of COVID-19', *Transforming Government: People, Process and Policy*, 15: 197–205. https://doi.org/10.1108/TG-09-2020-0269

UK Parliament (2023) 'Privileges Committee publish Boris Johnson written evidence ahead of oral evidence session', 21 March. Available at: https://committees.parliament.uk/committee/289/committee-of-privileges/news/194324/privileges-committee-publish-boris-johnson-written-evidence-ahead-of-oral-evidence-session/ (accessed 11 May 2023).

Youngs, R. (2020) 'Coronavirus: democracy is the missing link in EU recovery plans', *The Conversation*, 13 May. Available at: https://theconversation.com/coronavirus-democracy-is-the-missing-link-in-eu-recovery-plans-138442 (accessed 19 May 2023).

1

The epidemic as a life-event: epidemicity and epidemic form

Lina Minou, James Wilson and Daniel Herron

Everyday life and other conditions of normality were affected to such an extent during the coronavirus (COVID-19) pandemic that it seemed to many that they were living through a quite exceptional situation. However, a look to medical history quickly reminds us that, while what was experienced seemed exceptional to many, the sudden onset of an infectious disease that led to widespread and rapid restructuring of social possibilities was not unique. Epidemic diseases have emerged and re-emerged throughout history and they are imprinted in our cultural memory.[1]

Medical history points not only to the ordinariness of epidemics, their matter-of-factness, but also to the ordinary, regular patterns according to which they occur. With regard to the former, what makes epidemic diseases ordinary, epidemiologically speaking, is that the conditions for their occurrence are always already in place: new viruses will emerge, known viruses will mutate to pose threats, and pathogenic conditions – usually related to the broader eco-social environment and the organisation of our living – will materialise. The medical historian Frank Snowden (2008) had long warned against viewing them as something conquered or a thing of the past, and other scholars have warned against the hubristic attitude of doing so (Garrett, 2018). With regard to the latter, medical history teaches us that the recurrence of epidemics and their shock value have led to certain tropes in the way we talk about them, the way we expect them to develop and come to a close, and in the narratives we tell about them. Epidemics, that is, have a form.

Charles Rosenberg, writing in 1989, recognised this form as drama and went on to propose a model of dramaturgic logic in the way they unfold: 'epidemics start at a moment in time, proceed on a stage limited in space and duration, follow a plot line of increasing and revelatory tension, move to a crisis of individual and collective character, then drift toward closure' (Rosenberg, 1989: 2).

Epidemics, Rosenberg posits, proceed according to certain stages, initially 'progressive revelation' and 'recognition' of the event followed by coping strategies and closure. At the heart of Rosenberg's scheme lies intelligibility. There is no ambiguity with regard to what occurs. He notes that unlike other aspects of biological history that can proceed imperceptibly until 'discovered' by historians, epidemics are 'highly visible' phenomena (Rosenberg, 1989: 1–2). This underlies the predictability of their development which progresses along a pattern of *beginning-middle-end*. Other scholars have pointed to their formulaic structure: there are repetitive tropes, images, characters and storylines along which we talk about epidemics, and arguably in the way we experience them (Wald, 2008). The literary form of epidemic disease is no coincidence. David Steel, whose 1981 essay essentially establishes a literary canon, remarks that: 'epidemic diseases ... share with works of literature an inherent structure, an aetiology, rising from an onset, through a climax to a decline and an ending' (Steel, 1981: 107).

This affinity may be 'inherent', to a degree, but it is also confirmed as such by the way we look at epidemics. Paul Slack aptly notices that the long heritage of texts that chronicled their various occurrences through time themselves followed an archetype:

> One can never be entirely sure about the extent to which chroniclers of epidemics concentrated on social dislocation, the failure of doctors, flights to and from religion, rumours of poisoned wells, and similar phenomena simply because Thucydides and later writers down to Defoe taught them to look for them. (Slack, 1992: 9)

The textual heritage of epidemics taught us to look for certain patterns in their unfolding: recurring characters such as the 'patient zero', stories of infectiousness, suspicion towards possible carriers and so on. These were consolidated in repetition; by the practice of specifically looking to epidemics in the past and recognising these features. Scholars were guided to this by their attention-drawing aspect. As the historian Margaret Pelling observes, in the historiographical record there is a disparity of attention with regard to epidemic and endemic disease. Endemic disease, the regular cause of morbidity and mortality in a given area, tends, she says, to be considered normal and thus neglected. Epidemic disease, on the other hand, is dramatic and tends to hold our attention (Pelling, 2020: 294–295).

The insights offered above, are the product of analysis and thus derive from externalised perspectives. They are thoughts about the phenomenon 'from above', or from a physical and conceptual distance, or after the fact. They also consciously draw upon a specified written culture. They do not reflect the global aspects of epidemics. In the context of the current pandemic, scholars have revisited those models and tropes, questioning and revising them. Felicity Callard, writing from a human geography perspective, highlights how Rosenberg's model posits unities that are not as stable as implied: 'Rosenberg, in offering a dramaturgical logic to describe epidemic time, not only establishes a stage, but a particular sequencing of beginning, middle, and end. Any dramaturgical logic installs an imagined point from which the observer watches a plot line develop and, then, perhaps, resolve' (Callard, 2020: 728).

Proposing a different vantage point, what she calls 'thinking from the sickbed', Callard asks instead 'what kind of observation is possible when one is deeply entangled in what is unfolding' (Callard, 2020: 728). Her work takes two major public-initiated themes that originated within the context of the pandemic. One is the naming of the extended form of a COVID infection, that is, 'long COVID'. Callard notes that the particular phrase was a patient-bestowed name rather than one ascribed by medical professionals and that choice of the adjective 'long' – rather than any other term that would imply 'post' COVID – entails the undoing of temporal linearity and also of externally imposed time frames into the discussion of disease (Callard, 2020). The very term 'long COVID' complicates the sequence of *beginning-middle-end* of the pandemic itself.

The other theme concerns sufferers of chronic conditions, particularly Myalgic Encephalomyelitis/Chronic Fatigue Syndrome (ME/CFS), who recognised in the symptoms of long COVID similarities with the reality they have been experiencing for many years and which has been largely unnoticed or downplayed. The visibility of long COVID afforded visibility of their condition and this, remarks Callard, upsets the temporality of a pandemic narrative by allowing us to imagine a group of people who have essentially been waiting, in a sense, for the pandemic in order for their own concerns to become perceivable and to be given proper attention in the public and the scientific eye (Callard, 2020: 732). Thus, this 'collective thinking from the sickbed' has 'disturbed common epidemiological and medical means of adjudicating illness time' (Callard, 2020: 737). Instead of the linear conventions of medical science, whereby assigning severity and acuteness or chronicity also assigns valuations of suffering and of time, we are left with a 'difficult' temporality where 'different patients inhabit different temporal horizons, different narrative scripts, different histories, different experiences of duration' (Callard, 2020: 737).

Other scholars argue that we do not only need a look into epidemics from a different vantage point, but nothing short of a deconstruction of the models that circumscribe them. The historian Richard Keller notes how 'limiting' Rosenberg's dramaturgy is, because 'to circumscribe the pandemic with such a narrative device is to make it discrete rather than one facet of a broader experience of late capitalist modernity, or of peak Anthropocene' (Langstaff, 2020: para. 19 of 66). Guillaume Lachenal and Gaëtan Thomas argued for 'emancipat[ing] the historical narration of epidemics from a set of literary tropes cemented by centuries of intertextuality' (Lachenal and Thomas, 2020: 671). Looking to the multifaceted perspectives developed within African studies on the afterlives of pandemics, they reach a conceptual framework that rejects their notion as 'events oriented towards their own closure' and proposes instead their viewing as 'unsettling, seemingly endless, periods during which life has to be recomposed' (Lachenal and Thomas, 2020: 672). Lachenal and Thomas draw also on Jeremy Greene's and Dora Vargha's (2020) reflection on the elusive endings of pandemics and on the history of the AIDS epidemic, which leads to a reversal of Rosenberg's definition of the epidemic from 'event' into 'trend' (Lachenal and Thomas, 2020: 680). Their perspective allows for no fixed points, either of ending or beginnings. They observe that the African experience is characterised by 'copresence of deep and recent epidemic pasts' and so epidemics are 'best understood (and experienced) as contemporary to previous ones, nested into one another, like Russian dolls' (Lachenal and Thomas, 2020: 682).

Such explorations allow us to consider causes, management, experiences through varied contexts, inclusive of global perspectives. They allow us to zero in on the inequality and disparity of experience within the same geographical area, the same social bounds. This is what is gained, for instance, by Callard's analysis and its questioning of the linear temporality in epidemics. Conversely, we can also expand our view from the regional and the specific to greater scales. However, there is also something to be lost. Opening the form of epidemics can open our eyes to complex global issues and patterns, such as broad or global health inequalities, or generalisable human behaviours, but it can also blind us to the significance of each event to an individual life. There is a danger that the visibility of what is grander, complex and encompassing will come at the expense of what is single and singularised.

In this discussion we reflect on the relation between the intellectual constructs of the epidemic phenomenon and its meaning as an occurrence within an individual life. We begin by acknowledging that certain elements of epidemic discourse have a basis in disease behaviour and as such they cannot be denied. To be specific, a defining aspect of epidemics is their emergence which, at the most basic level, is a breaking off with the extant public health conditions in a given area. Compared to endemic disease, epidemics have the capacity to surprise us, they are unanticipated or unusual – that is, in some manner they do *rise*. This suggests that a basic pattern of arise-rise-fall does circumscribe epidemics, even though in actuality those specified points can be elusive. We further suggest that in the context of the current pandemic we have conceptually followed that pattern, guided not only through pervasive intellectual constructs, but mainly through the information and data-driven culture within which we have experienced the coronavirus pandemic unfolding.

This pattern, on its own, does not do justice to the meaning of an epidemic for an individual as a life-event. This much has been shown by the corrective views offered by recent scholarly discussion. Callard's analysis has shown us that if epidemics are drama there is a multiplicity of other dramas enfolded into the main one, with different rhythms and structures. Lachenal and Thomas (2020) have made us aware that there is no event–aftermath dyad; that life becomes recomposed exactly as the seemingly endless period of a pandemic goes on. Our discussion proposes that a way to unveil the separate, individual rhythms of the enfolded dramas of the epidemic is to consider them as 'events' in the specific way posited by phenomenological theory.

Our premise is the following: (1) the defining element of an epidemic is its emergence, its onset: where it peaks or how it ends are important structural elements, but not necessary to define it. Indeed, epidemics come into being once proclaimed as such. (2) This emergence or onset is recognised in specified ways in epidemiological terms, it signifies a breaking off from extant conditions. This means something unsettles the norms and thus is extraordinary in some way. (3) Emergence and extraordinariness are two prominent conceptual threads that allow us to understand epidemics. However, we need a separate account regarding what makes something extraordinary epidemiologically versus what makes it extraordinary in the context of lived experience. These two are qualitatively different concepts. We suggest, therefore, that within epidemicity, which follows a priori aetiological and explanatory frameworks, various epidemic life-events transpire that are truly original in that they are neither anticipated nor fully explained by pre-existing frameworks. To do justice, then, to the complexity of the several manifestations of the epidemic reality, we need an equally complex conceptual framework, one that is co-produced by historical and philosophical insight.

Senses of 'event'

We talk of epidemics as extraordinary events. To formally declare one requires making use of the very term. A PHEIC (Public Health Emergency of International Concern), such as the current COVID-19 pandemic, is an 'extraordinary event that may constitute a public health risk to other states through international spread of disease and to potentially require a coordinated international response' (WHO, 2005).[2] The guidance describes a situation that is serious, sudden, unusual or unexpected. The term 'event' here is being used in the common, everyday sense of 'significant occurrence'. In this sense, 'extraordinary' suggests a breaking off with conditions of normality as they are understood in a given situation. The epidemic as it happens to an individual, though, and its meaning, cannot be exhausted in that factually defined occurrence. We need to distinguish between these two notions of an epidemic. We will do this by defining 'event', following phenomenological theorist Claude Romano, as the reconfiguration of possibility in one's life that is truly original and refers only to itself. By contrast, epidemicity rests on factual conditions and contexts that pre-exist and explain it.

Epidemicity

The *Dictionary of Epidemiology* defines epidemic as follows:

> EPIDEMIC: The occurrence in a community or region of cases of an illness, specific health-related behavior, or other health-related events clearly in excess of normal expectancy. The community or region and the period in which the cases occur must be specified precisely. The number of cases indicating the presence of an epidemic varies according to the agent, size, and type of population exposed; previous experience or lack of exposure to the disease; and time and place of occurrence. Epidemicity is thus relative to usual frequency of the disease in the same area, among the specified population, at the same season of the year. (Porta et al., 2014: 93)

According to the above, what seems to define epidemic disease – where the extraordinariness lies – is this capacity to unsettle the usual conditions of public health in a given area. It is not about morbidity or mortality per se, but their excess in relation to existing norms. Thus, epidemicity is of relative originality in that this always depends on the state of conditions that it comes to unsettle.

This breaking off with normalcy conditions, however these are defined, *is* the rising of the epidemic. The identification of that moment in time may fluctuate. Some may choose to equate the beginning with first recorded cases, others with first acute hospitalisations. Other perspectives may defer the beginning still further and argue that the real start occurs at the microscopic level, when the infection actually takes place. Depending on the scale used, the beginning of the epidemic may be fixed or flexible, but it is always accessible as a point in time. This is because the beginning of the epidemic is necessarily linked to the aetiological framework of disease. Even if we follow an open form, we cannot do completely away with a point of origin, a point of emergence. Even in regions of repeated outbreaks, we can recognise a trend, but within this trend it would still be possible to identify beginnings of separate cycles of epidemicity. This is the essential condition of an epidemic: that it rises and because of this it is expected to fall. This is apprehensible in the specified conditions of epidemiology. It is not the same as recognition, though.

The recognition that Rosenberg identifies as stage one of an epidemic is not an unaided, immediate and unmediated grasping of reality. Both an epidemic and a pandemic require a formal announcement to be perceived as such. In a sense, then, the very naming of a disease as 'epidemic' makes it so in an instant of performative language. This is more pronounced in modern societies where death has retreated in visibility and happens largely out of the public eye (Mellor, 1992; Mellor and Shilling, 1993). Following the pronouncement, recognition then proceeds along evidence that nowadays is more and more quantitative in nature, such as death numbers, hospitalisations, the rate of infection, and so on. We do not wish to draw too bold a distinction line here: epidemics in pre-modern societies were understood by morbidity and mortality numbers. However, it is notable that in plague writing of the Renaissance, for instance, the medical historian Margaret Healy recognises two major themes: one of 'supernatural or natural explanation as to the "how" and "why" of the affliction' and a second of 'the eyewitness account that details signs, symptoms, and the effect of epidemic in society in visual and moral terms' (Healy, 2001: 61–62). In a way, we still bear witness to the effects of the epidemic through the personal stories that feature in the news and which give shape to the notion of infectiousness. However, for the most part we follow the epidemic through data and graphs. We interpret and visualise epidemics in a particular way, mainly through the wave graph, which is itself laden with metaphorical and symbolic meaning beyond its objective values (Eyler, 2002; Jones and Helmreich, 2020). Epidemic data reach us with added, expert, interpretation. Hence in modern-day epidemics, the recognition that one is living through an epidemic is progressively a mediated act, albeit one that is punctuated by the deaths and illness of friends and family members.

What is more, the data culture surrounding epidemics does not simply describe the phenomenon. Rather, it creates anticipation spurred by our aim to predict the course of the disease. But our anticipation is not necessarily met. For instance, the crisis, the peak of an epidemic, can be theoretically located on the fixed, and determinable, point of greatest number of cases or excess deaths. As we reach a point that data sketch out as critical, this may also be deferred by conversations that look to the future; to another wave, to the possibility of a number that is bigger yet. The same happens with resolution. We can fix it on the ending point of measures being lifted, or case numbers falling, but, as happened with the official date of lifting restrictions in the UK, this point can be set and then invalidated – while the falling number can turn out as too fragile a factor. Indeed, as Greene and Vargha reflect: 'at their best, epidemic endings are a form of relief for the mainstream "we" that can pick up the pieces and reconstitute a normal life. At their worst, epidemic endings are a form of collective amnesia, transmuting the disease that remains into merely someone else's problem' (Greene and Vargha, 2020: para. 27 of 31).

In other words, as the drama of the epidemic unfolds, we do not proceed with clarity from one stage to another, but we are *waiting* for each one of these stages. The absence of a fixed ending is immaterial in this respect. The essential form through which we discuss epidemics creates waiting for, and anticipation of, an 'aftermath', a continuously projected future. This future is neither truly authentic nor solely based on the particular epidemic that happens now. It is shaped by our collective epidemic past and the way this is revived through experience, direct comparison with past epidemics, through interpretation, and through its preservation in text. In sum, it can be said that epidemicity is of relative originality or exceptionality, of more or less established form, and of mediated intelligibility. More than that, it is impersonal.

Epidemic as life-event

An epidemic occurs within a community, but is not assigned to anyone specifically, it befalls all of us. The epidemic as life-*event*, by contrast, occurs in my own life, spells out a particular reconfiguration of my possibilities and brings me closer to an 'unanticipated future' that makes sense for me specifically. Following Claude Romano's evential hermeneutics, the event concentrates the following aspects:

> An event is truly original, in that it is not exhausted in the fact in which it occurred and cannot be anticipated and explained by a priori frameworks. An event truly *arises* in an individual life.
>
> An event reconfigures the sum of my possibility and thus presents me with a future that is unanticipated and is made possible only due to the event's arising.
>
> An event is a hermeneutical phenomenon; it leads me to understand myself differently in light of the future it brings with it. The event arises with the full cargo of its possibilities, it is not retrospective judgment.
>
> Finally, the event has the capacity to singularize me, the traversing of events in my life, and the precise way they have reconfigured my possibility and will continue to do so, give me my biography.
> (Romano, 2009)

Accordingly, then, to experience the epidemic as a life-event is a profoundly original phenomenon. Societies can prepare for an epidemic and can make use of historical insight to do so. Nothing can prepare a person for living through the event. Elizabeth Rourke, a US medical doctor who wrote about her personal experience of the pandemic, remarks in her reflection: 'I never saw this coming when I went into medicine' (Rourke, 2020: 2185).

The epidemic considered as a life-event is constituted in the reconfiguration of possibility that is referred solely to its arising. Consider, for instance, a person who changes profession due to the way they are influenced by the COVID-related epidemic, choosing to enter the healthcare sector. Conversely, think of someone impacted by long COVID who cannot return to a job they loved and saw as part of their identity, or someone who may have lost the opportunity for life-altering medical treatment due to the pandemic's impact on medical services. For the people involved in those cases, what led to their situation – such as strained services, social and working conditions, specificities of disease susceptibility, specific infectiousness conditions in their area of living – is relevant, but never sufficient to fully account for their experience.

Many other life-events can be recognised as well that can be linked either to infectious conditions or to the living conditions that the infection introduced, such as quarantine and isolation. Again, the frameworks that explain the necessity of these living conditions can never account for the 'why' of the personal event. Those who experience the infection as a life-event can neither anticipate nor prepare for it. In Romano's words: 'the *event* of an illness, as it happens unsubstitutably to an *advenant* by reconfiguring his essential possibilities, his world, and by bringing him to *understand himself* differently, is rigorously *without a why* and *happens "because it happens"*. It is itself its own *origin*' (Romano, 2009: 58).

That the event happens 'unsubstitutably' to someone denotes the dynamic relation between event and the one who goes through it (the 'advenant' in Romano's words). Specifically, that meaning is created in the interaction between event and 'advenant'. Event, then, is no effect or aftermath: something that impacts upon and changes an already formed and stable self. Romano posits that events give us our biography in that what happens to us singularises us. To illustrate the point, not all those who suffer from long COVID traverse the same event. This is due not only to the diverse clinical manifestations of the condition, but also to the different histories of those who suffer from it; differences that were shaped by the events that shaped those different histories themselves. That is, each advenant, to use Romano's term, arrives at the long COVID event having traversed different other events in their own personal history. The long COVID event spells a specific reconfiguration of possibility that makes sense to each one in particular. Hence, unlike epidemicity, we cannot speak of a group event, not even one rooted in a common medical context. There is commonality in such experiences, but not necessarily *sharedness*.

The life-event defines its own temporality. Events, as posited by Romano, are instantiated according to what has already transpired and with the full cargo of the possibilities they carry. In this case, life-events transpire according to the already proclaimed epidemic and instantly reveal the future they spell for each advenant. This evential 'future' is neither consequence nor aftermath. It is not a matter of time difference, but a qualitatively different 'after' that is assuredly perceived exactly as the event arises. Rather, *it is* the arising of the event. This future is truly authentic, as nothing prepares for it, or anticipates it, other than the event itself. What is more, though not precisely correlated to the unfolding of the epidemic itself, the evential future is rooted in the factual occurrence of the event itself and, as such, is separate from a collective epidemic past.

The life-event is essentially an interpretative act, in light of which the advenant reaches a different understanding of themselves and, as such, cannot be captured in quantitively defined time. For this reason, the life-event does not correlate to the development stages of the epidemiological occurrence. This is the reason why people experience lapses between formal announcements and their own personal realisations. Elizabeth Rourke, for instance, describes how she went from a point where ordinary life remained uninterrupted, to seeing fewer patients in the first weeks of March 2020 and finally the moment she understands everything as 'changed' (Rourke, 2020: 2184). This lapse is also discernible in the many references to the 'old life', the life before COVID, that abound and are being used not retrospectively, but *as* the pandemic unfolds. In Rourke's account, for example, 'I never saw this coming' is complemented by reflection on the already changed self: '[M]y old life, 2 weeks ago, feels like it happened to another person' (Rourke, 2020: 2185). Realisations such as the one cited by Rourke above, are not externally imposed. The intelligibility of the life-event is truly unmediated.

In sum, then, we can identify life-events as phenomena of profound originality, of unmediated intelligibility and of no established form – though not form-less. The originality of the event means a stark difference is created between its arising or its absence. This difference derives solely from the event. Those who experience the epidemic-as-event are confronted with 'futures' of reconfigured possibility. These futures are to be found in the interpretative function of events: in their capacity to present us with different articulations of possibility within our life, whether these have positive or negative valence, and lead us to redefine ourselves. In this respect, we must refine our notion of people experiencing different durations within the unfolding of a main social drama. To experience the epidemic-as-event is not a question of different rhythm but of a different sense of immediacy. It is not witnessing the 'progressive revelation' of Rosenberg's drama, it is an immediate recognition of changed possibilities. It is to be 'entangled into what is unfolding' but in an individual rather than a collective manner. It is to acknowledge that people live through profound change irrespective of how epidemicity itself develops or concludes.

Co-presence and contemporaneity

Not everyone experiences the epidemic as a life-event. This is true for any given geographical setting, whether the memory of past epidemics is still vivid or not. The event-ness of the epidemic does not rest on originality in the sense of being novel or unprecedented. Event-ness itself, as defined by Romano, does not depend on a firm subject, an experiencing self, who gives meaning to what occurs in life. Rather, it is co-produced in an interaction between advenant and event. In turn, this signifies that even people who have gone through epidemic cycles, or have experienced them as 'trend' may also experience one of these cycles as life-event, in the sense described here. More than that, it means that as we go through the current pandemic, and as we slowly and uncertainly move away from it, various individual versions of it have been, and are, co-present. There are people who grapple with the newly revealed futures of life-events, but these are also as dissimilar to each other as are the histories of the people experiencing them. This is because these histories, in turn, are produced by the sum of events in those individual lives and how these have shaped the advenant of this particular life-event. This may also signify an advenant who has already experienced a previous epidemic, or epidemics, or other life-events. By contrast, there are people who experience the epidemic as not eventful; neither original nor revealing.

It is then useful at this point to return to the concept of epidemic occurrences as 'nested' into one another as Lachenal and Thomas propose, but with certain modifications. The authors reached this description thinking of the recurrence of epidemics within a geographical region. However, we argue that it is not absolutely necessary for actual epidemics to occur in order for the epidemic past to be co-present with the unfolding epidemic. It can be made present through exegesis and the attempts at interpretation of the experience. The collective epidemic past may become 'nested' into the epidemiological occurrence through the authoritative texts that make up the genre of 'plague' writing, or may be raised through data comparison with epidemics of the past, or through the anticipation of the regularised stages of the epidemic. What is also 'nested' within epidemicity is the potential for epidemics-as-life-events. It is important to recognise the co-presence of those elements. It is also important, however, to distinguish between co-presence and contemporaneity.

To reiterate, epidemics materialise in an epidemiologically defined fact. Their actualisation as significant occurrences carries with it certain contextual elements that have been established intellectually through a combination of historical experience, historical insight, information, stories and comparative thinking. This, in a sense is the *en-present-ment* of an epidemic past. At the same time, the experience of an epidemic, or of several cycles of epidemics, always carries with it the potential for epidemics-as-life-events. These manifestations of the epidemic phenomenon are not exactly contemporaneous to each other. As illustrated above, contemporaneity between the social fact of the epidemic occurrence and the personal life-event is not possible as the event occurs according to its own temporality.

Recurrent epidemic outbreaks, and the way these may bring the epidemic past into being, may establish familiarity, but not contemporaneity. This is because meaning is created through the interaction between event and the one who goes through it. Even if an occurrence is unoriginal and unrevealing – in other words a non-event in Romano's terms – the difference between a past selfhood and a current selfhood, as this is shaped by the traversing of events, means also the clear apprehension of difference in terms of temporality. This is perhaps the most distinguishing insight that philosophy can afford us into the experience of epidemics. If we are to acknowledge the historicity of epidemics – their 'palimpsest-like structures and temporalities' (Lachenal and Thomas, 2020: 671) – we must also acknowledge how this may obscure the dynamic between events and those who go through them. Unlike the receptive nature of a palimpsest as medium, as surface that captures change without changing in itself, the bodies and selves that go through epidemics change constantly through events. Appreciating this helps account for change in the lives of people who go through an epidemic that does not derive from the particular way they are emplaced in the social drama – their social position, their health status, their vulnerability – but from their own capacity as evential beings.

Conclusion

Describing epidemics as social drama is not an obsolete analogy. It is a useful tool in understanding epidemics as long as we are conscious of its inherent limitations. What we need in order to understand the epidemic phenomenon is to attain to its complexity through a layered framework of thought that can include the multiplicity of experiences that characterise it. This framework has to include multiple senses of 'event' because this thought can alert us to different aspects of originality and thus to different ways of making meaning. Historical insight can alert us as to the commonality and the tropes of our experience. Philosophical insight can provide us with the language with which to express its uniqueness and distinctiveness. Different senses of 'event', the choice of describing it as 'bounded' or not, as defined epidemiologically or as seen in other disciplines, will allow the multiplicity of perspectives that we need. It will also afford us insights into the temporality(ies) of the phenomenon, which beyond being described as complex, are a major part of what differentiates the experience for those who supposedly live through it simultaneously. The closed, dramaturgic model proposed by Rosenberg, the open models that came to revise it, and the self-referential model of Romano, taken together, reveal what is characteristic about epidemics: they are neither ordinary (or normalised as endemic disease, for instance) nor extraordinary in themselves. Rather, they oscillate between ordinariness and originality. This carries capacity for different kinds of hermeneutics. To return to, and revise, Rosenberg's definition, an epidemic is both *'events* and a trend'. In light of this, there is not a given 'collective we' that can reprise normal life after the end of an epidemic. A 'collective we' needs to be constituted out of *collective stories*; constructed by facts, the broader socio-cultural contexts in which these facts occur, and our interpretation of them. A crucial place into this interpretation must be afforded into how *one's life-story* is shaped when traversing the experience of a life-event.

Notes

1 The definition of a pandemic is contested. Most definitions take a pandemic to be an epidemic that crosses international boundaries and occurs in a wide geographical area simultaneously. As de Campos (2020) examines, none of the standard definitions take severity to be a defining feature of pandemics, and some do not even require a pandemic to involve an infectious disease outbreak. The result is that the concept of pandemic can often be used in an unhelpfully broad way: communicable diseases that do not rise to a level of severity to threaten the need for emergency responses, or even non-communicable diseases such as obesity have sometimes been referred to as pandemics by the WHO. In this chapter, we are interested in epidemics of communicable disease that are of wide geographical spread and which do reach a level of severity that could require an emergency response. We take it to be uncontroversial that COVID-19 presented such a case.

2 A PHEIC, being an operative term, is narrower than our usual understanding of an epidemic. However, the term does serve to showcase the unexpectedness of an epidemic occurring relative to the normal conditions over a given area. Additionally, we make use of the term here because it represents a formal point of 'emergence' or 'beginning' without anticipating an end. Once announced, a PHEIC is reviewed every three months and can be maintained for long periods, see for example polio-related PHEIC, in place since 2014, at: www.who.int/news/item/21-05-2021-statement-following-the-twenty-eighth-ihr-emergency-committee-for-polio

References

Callard, F. (2020) 'Epidemic time: thinking from the sickbed', *Bulletin of the History of Medicine*, 94(4): 727–743. https://doi.org/10.1353/bhm.2020.0093

de Campos, T. C. (2020) 'The traditional definition of pandemics, its moral conflations, and its practical implications: a defense of conceptual clarity in global health laws and policies', *Cambridge Quarterly of Healthcare Ethics*, 29(2): 205–217. https://doi.org/10.1017/S0963180119001002

Eyler, J. M. (2002) 'Constructing vital statistics: Thomas Rowe Edmonds and William Farr, 1835–1845', *Soz Präventivmed*, 47: 6–13.

Garrett, L. (2018) 'Human arrogance and epidemics', *The Lancet*, 391(10123): 827–828. https://doi.org/10.1016/S0140-6736(18)30433-1

Greene, J. A. and Vargha, D. (2020) 'How epidemics end', *Boston Review*, 30 June. Available at: https://bostonreview.net/articles/jeremy-greene-dora-vargha-how-epidemics-end-or-dont/ (accessed 18 April 2023).

Healy, M. (2001) *Fictions of Disease in Early Modern England: Bodies, Plagues and Politics*, Basingstoke: Palgrave Macmillan.

Jones, D. S. and Helmreich, S. (2020) 'The shape of epidemics', *Boston Review*, 26 June. Available at: www.bostonreview.net/articles/david-shumway-jones-stefan-helmreich-epidemic-waves/ (accessed 18 April 2023).

Lachenal, G. and Thomas, G. (2020) 'Epidemics have lost the plot', *Bulletin of the History of Medicine*, 94(4): 670–689. https://doi.org/10.1353/bhm.2020.0089

Langstaff, A. (2020) 'Pandemic narratives and the historian', *Los Angeles Review of Books*, 18 May. Available at: www.lareviewofbooks.org/article/pandemic-narratives-and-the-historian/ (accessed 18 April 2023).

Mellor, P. A. (1992) 'Death in high modernity: the contemporary presence and absence of death', *The Sociological Review*, 40(1): 11–30. https://doi.org:10.1111/j.1467-954X.1992.tb03384.x

Mellor, P. A. and Shilling, C. (1993) 'Modernity, self-identity and the sequestration of death', *Sociology*, 27(3): 411–431. https://doi.org/10.1177/0038038593027003005

Pelling, M. (2020) ' "Bosom vipers": endemic versus epidemic disease', *Centaurus*, 62(2): 294–301. https://doi.org/10.1111/1600-0498.12297

Porta, M. S. et al. (eds) (2014) *A Dictionary of Epidemiology*, International Epidemiological Association (6th edn), Oxford: Oxford University Press.

Romano, C. (2009) *Event and World* (trans. S. Mackinlay), New York: Fordham University Press.

Rosenberg, C. E. (1989) 'What is an epidemic? AIDS in historical perspective', *Daedalus*, 118(2): 1–17. Available at: www.jstor.org/stable/20025233

Rourke, E. J. (2020) 'Waiting', *New England Journal of Medicine*, 382(23): 2184–2185. https://doi.org/10.1056/NEJMp2007073

Slack, P. (1992) 'Introduction', in T. Ranger and P. Slack (eds) *Epidemics and Ideas: Essays on the Historical Perception of Pestilence*, Cambridge: Cambridge University Press, 1–20.

Snowden, F. M. (2008) 'Emerging and reemerging diseases: a historical perspective', *Immunological Reviews*, 225(1): 9–26. https://doi.org/10.1111/j.1600-065X.2008.00677.x

Steel, D. (1981) 'Plague writing: from Boccaccio to Camus', *Journal of European Studies*, 11(42): 88–110.

Wald, P. (2008) *Contagious Cultures, Carriers, and the Outbreak Narrative*, Durham, NC: Duke University Press.

World Health Organization (2005) *International Health Regulations* (3rd edn). Available at: www.who.int/publications/i/item/9789241580496

2

Relationships were a casualty when pandemic ethics and everyday clinical ethics collided

Caroline Redhead, Anna Chiumento, Sara Fovargue, Heather Draper and Lucy Frith

The young woman who had gone into premature labour had just returned home after visiting family overseas. The UK rules at that time required her to self-isolate for two weeks after she got back, and she gave birth before that period of quarantine had ended. Hospital infection prevention and control measures meant that, having delivered her baby, she had to stay, alone, in her specifically designated accommodation. She was not allowed to visit her baby on the ward, despite having twice tested negative for Covid-19. Appeals by her baby's healthcare team to make an exception for her were unsuccessful. The baby died a week later – and only when the baby was dying, were the rules relaxed. Then, for the first and only time in its short life, were the baby's mother and father able to be together with their child.[1]

Impossibly difficult experiences like this characterised the data collected as part of our 'Reset Ethics' research, which explored the everyday ethical challenges of reconfiguring (resetting) England's NHS maternity and paediatrics services during the coronavirus (COVID-19) pandemic. This 'resetting' created a unique context in which it became critical to consider how ethical considerations did (and should) underpin decisions about integrating infection control measures into the routine practice of healthcare. Healthcare professionals told us that the ethical challenges they encountered were often embedded in changes to working practices intended to keep them safe, and to protect hospital communities from COVID-19 infection. However, the impact of changes to working practices mandated by infection prevention and control measures reduced healthcare professionals' ability to 'care' for their patients, where care is understood as embracing the interpersonal relationships between the patient (and their family) and the healthcare provider. The importance of these interpersonal relationships is a key aspect of our data: offering care within a supportive relationship between healthcare professionals, their patients and (particularly in the context of maternity and children's services) a child's family. This was experienced as an ethically important dimension of healthcare delivery, and an essential component of patient-centred care. The ethical challenges our participants discussed were linked to the impact on these interpersonal relationships of the mandatory, non-negotiable infection prevention and control measures imposed during the pandemic.

It is this focus on infection prevention within healthcare settings that situates the puzzle that we address in our chapter. It is a puzzle because, at first blush, it seems entirely reasonable – and ethical – to focus on infection control measures in order to keep staff and patients safe in healthcare settings. It is surely imperative to take all necessary steps to keep hospital communities safe, for reasons that are obvious. Our findings suggest, however, that, although they protected healthcare staff and patients from COVID-19, infection, prevention and control measures, such as social distancing rules, visiting restrictions and the requirement to wear personal protective equipment (PPE), actually caused significant *harm* by creating barriers to interpersonal interaction and engagement in everyday healthcare practices. Infection prevention and control measures were not negotiable: the caring relationships *had* to give way. While, in our view, healthcare professionals and patients alike understood the need for strict infection control measures in the early acute phase of the pandemic, this changed during later waves of infection. At this point, we will argue, a focus on *relationships* would have helped to inform decision-making. The harms of refusing a new parent access to a sick baby despite her having tested negative for COVID-19, for example, might have been mitigated by allowing the parents and the healthcare professionals to discuss and agree a safe, fair and less harmful interpretation of the rules for that particular circumstance.

In this chapter, we situate our participants' reflections in a discussion about the importance of relationships and their significance in a healthcare context. The chapter proceeds as follows. In the first section, we introduce our study, touching briefly on the methodology adopted and the challenges we encountered. We next draw on our data to highlight the vital importance and value of the relationships that many healthcare professionals felt were central to the 'family-centred' maternity and paediatric services that were our focus. The theoretical underpinnings of a logic of relationality are then described, and we consider how our data support the importance of such a logic in the healthcare context. In the following section, we discuss the risks of disrupting relationships, considering moral distress as one of the possible consequences of damaging the human *caring* relationships within which healthcare is embedded.

In concluding, we contend that an explicit attention to relationships is required to provide effective support to healthcare professionals in responding both to the everyday stresses and strains of working in healthcare, *and* to the extraordinary impacts of a public health emergency. Progress towards achieving this will be made by adopting an approach to decision-making that foregrounds the importance of relational engagement.

The 'Reset Ethics' project in context: the background to the empirical research

The effects of the COVID-19 pandemic on the NHS have been profound. The cycle of starting, suspending and restarting routine services has been ongoing for over three years at the time of writing in 2023, and, with the impact of new variants of COVID-19, continues. This process of 'resetting' has required consideration of how best to (re)organise healthcare services and (re)allocate resources so that COVID *and* non-COVID healthcare services can continue in tandem. New kinds of ethical issues and dilemmas have undoubtedly arisen as decision-makers have had to continually (re)assess the best way to balance individual access to healthcare services and the continued protection of hospital communities and the wider public from COVID-19.

In April 2020, healthcare providers were asked by the government in England to step up non-COVID-19 urgent services as soon as possible (Stevens and Pritchard, 2020). The key question then facing healthcare providers was *how* to reset these services, some of which had been required to cease the previous month. Guidelines and policies, which were rapidly developed to underpin the acute coronavirus response, had drawn on existing ethical frameworks, and posited pandemic-specific approaches to decision-making in anticipated worst-case scenarios.[2] These documents, however, demonstrated little attention to the need to balance responses to the pandemic *with* the concurrent provision of non-pandemic healthcare, such as maternity and paediatric services. The central aim of our research was to consider *how*, in that context, decision-makers had understood and attended to the new kinds of ethical issues and dilemmas that were unique to the 'resetting' of everyday healthcare practices and process.

To investigate which ethical values were relevant, and to what extent they featured in guidance about the reorganisation of maternity and paediatric services, we conducted an analysis of the policies and processes current between April 2020 and March 2021. Our review asked, 'Which ethical values (explicitly or implicitly) guided decision-making in non-COVID-19 paediatric surgery and maternity services during the initial NHS reset in England?' (Chiumento et al., 2021). We adopted a rapid review methodology, taking a comprehensive yet pragmatic approach to the searches, screening, analysis and appraisal of sources, and conducted a qualitative thematic synthesis of the included documents. We reviewed a diverse range of documents, such as government and hospital trust policies, statements and decision support tools; reports and statements from professional bodies and charitable organisations; and evidence reviews and commentaries in academic journals.

An interesting finding of the rapid review was that patternings of relationships were visible in numerous ways and were anchored in both the individual *and* organisational mutual dependencies and responsibilities that the pandemic has starkly highlighted. Relationality was implicit in inter-NHS organisational collaborations locally, regionally and nationally to coordinate continuity of care. There was also clear recognition of the ethical importance of acknowledging the adverse impact of the pandemic on caring and dependent relationships, while simultaneously attending to public safety. However, while the fundamental importance of relationships in healthcare practice was acknowledged, there was no meaningful engagement with the ways in which relationships might be valued in practice. It was this lack of attention to the value of relationships in the resetting of healthcare practice that, we argue, left the door open to the ethical difficulties experienced by our participants. The impact of many of the changed practices appeared to be particularly significant on the family and caring relationships inherent to our areas of focus: birthing partners in maternity care, and parents or carers in paediatric services.

The findings of the rapid review informed the design of the interview guides for the qualitative data collection in our Reset Ethics project, particularly the interviews with senior decision-makers in our participating NHS hospital Trusts. An important aim of these interviews was to tease out the ethical values guiding both the approach to decision-making and the justifications for the decisions made, whether implicit or explicit. We were also interested in the reasons for any disagreements, whether (and how) these were mediated, and the degree to which the decision was then successfully implemented. Interviews and focus group discussions with healthcare professionals sought to explore senior management decision-making from a different perspective. These interviews focused on the way(s) participants' working practices had to change to accommodate the resetting of paediatric and maternity services, and how clearly these changes, and the reasons for them, were communicated. We explored how participants felt about these changes and asked them to talk about any ethical challenges or difficulties they had experienced as a result.

Pandemic and everyday ethics in collision: the empirical research

Six NHS hospital Trusts took part in our study. From these, senior managers and healthcare professionals were recruited for interviews and to participate in focus group discussions. The recruitment period (from October 2020 to July 2021, inclusive) spanned the national and regional lockdowns imposed during repeated waves of COVID-19 infection in the UK (Institute for Government, 2022), which clearly placed heightened demands on healthcare management and clinical staff. As a result, recruitment was challenging across the whole study. A total of eleven senior managers (seven female and four male) took part, and we spoke to twenty-six healthcare professionals (twenty female and six male) – doctors (nine), nurses (twelve) and midwives (five).

Having completed the individual interviews, we looked more closely at the ethical challenges described by the interview participants in focus groups with healthcare professionals. The initial thematic analysis of the interview data had identified the prevalence of reference to moral distress in healthcare professionals' accounts. Moral distress is the psychological, emotional and physiological suffering that people sometimes experience when they act in ways that are inconsistent with deeply held ethical values, principles or commitments: 'moral distress arises when one knows the right thing to do, but institutional constraints make it nearly impossible to pursue the right course of action' (Jameton, 1984: 6).[3]

In July 2021, we convened a focus group with six clinical psychologists in order to explore the finding about moral distress in more detail. The psychologists' role pre-pandemic had been to offer support to patients and families dealing with difficult clinical situations (such as end of life decisions), and to help them come to terms with what was happening. During the pandemic, however, these clinical psychologists agreed that their support had increasingly been sought by healthcare professionals *for themselves*, rather than for their patients. This was a notable change to their pre-pandemic practice. The focus group discussion explored in detail how the clinical psychologists had been asked to support their colleagues. In this discussion it became apparent that the moral distress described arose from the institutional constraints preventing the enactment of human relationships in the way participants' personal and professional ethical codes would usually direct. Thus, this moral distress had its roots in, and was a significant legacy for healthcare professionals of, the changed healthcare practices – such as social distancing – intended to have a protective effect from the physical effects of SARS-CoV-2 infection.

To explore these implications of changed working practices in more depth, we considered with further healthcare professional focus groups the changes that they would *not* want to see normalised, and why. Following an expression of interest from a senior physiotherapist, we recruited focus group participants (n = 13) from a team of paediatric physiotherapists spanning a range of specialties, including palliative care, serious burns and traumatic brain injuries. Two discussion groups were planned, however, due to a resurgence of COVID-19, shift patterns and staff holidays, dates for focus group discussions were difficult to coordinate. Ultimately only one focus group was held (with n = 5 participants) and a further two participants attended individual interviews. In the discussions, participants considered the ethical challenges raised by the practices about which they felt most uncomfortable, worked through what had made them challenging, and told us what (if they could choose) they felt would provide appropriate ethics support for them and their colleagues in the future.

The views and experiences of members of the public were also explored in focus groups with participants who had either had direct involvement with maternity or paediatric services during the pandemic, or had some prior experience of, or interest in, public involvement in NHS Trust decision-making. Recruitment to these focus groups was undertaken primarily by social media, through contacts made with local Trust patient partnership organisations, such as Maternity Voices Partnership (MVP),[4] Healthwatch[5] and Patient and Public Involvement (PPI) groups. Five focus groups were held in May and June 2021, involving a total of twenty-six participants. Participants were located geographically close to our participating Trusts; some had been patients at participating Trusts and some at other hospitals.

Our findings: making visible the importance of relationships

Our empirical data reflected the importance of relationships in various ways. Senior managers, for example, discussed the benefits of increased collaboration between Trusts and other organisations both regionally and more locally:

> So COVID has brought the system closer together. And we've been meeting with our like-minded partners on a weekly basis since COVID, started. (Chief Medical Officer, Foundation Trust)

> And I think it really has changed the way we view the local maternity and neonatal service now because previously they were suddenly you know, they were a nice add on and somewhere where you went and spoke to friendly faces and kind of shared, but through this we've

really come together and we've started to you know discuss cases and make joint decisions and look at us much more as one in the sector. (Head of Midwifery, District General Hospital [DGH])[6]

Interestingly, though, tensions between offering mutual aid and supporting staff in their 'home' hospital raised challenging questions:

> So we had a mutual aid request, can we give some of our masks to the adult hospital? Potentially, what that meant was, we wouldn't have masks for our staff. So I got, I got one body saying, essentially hide some in a cupboard, say no, we need to protect our own staff. I've got another body saying, how can you possibly leave all the people in another hospital at risk, knowing we've got some in the cupboard? And I couldn't form a view … to protect my own, which is really selfish. Or do I benefit the wider health economy, which I think ethically is the right thing to do? So we took [it] to the ethics committee … and they came back with, we have a duty to help the health economy, we have a duty to share. (Deputy Chief Nurse, Children's Hospital)

As well as discussing the benefits of regional collaboration, participants were positive about increasing collaboration within large hospital settings:

> There's probably a slight culture change … we've got four divisions, I wouldn't say there is competition between the divisions, but they're discrete business units. And we have league tables between them, etc. With the pandemic, it was being very much more of sharing of resource and supporting each other. And I absolutely want to keep that culture going. (Chief Operating Officer, NHS Foundation Trust)

Our data showed that the focus on the safety of all hospital staff during COVID-19 encouraged the maintenance of relationships in different ways, particularly the use of video-conferencing and other technology-based solutions where possible: 'But you could do it via Zoom. And we, we developed a whole new method of doing chief execs briefings, of communicating to staff, so on and so forth. So I think that was good. And we got good feedback from that' (Deputy Chief Medical Officer, Foundation Trust).

The limitations of 'electronic relationships' were often noted too:

> I think having things on over computers are really difficult, isn't it? And I think there's a lot of soft communication has been lost within

the organisation and a lot of, from a personal perspective, and I know from the Chief Nurse's perspective, we used to walk around the organisation a lot more. Now I just sit in front of a screen. (Executive medical director, DGH)

Recognising the challenges that physically remote leadership can engender, some participants described creative solutions to support staff morale. Initiatives that were intended to support a feeling of 'all-being-in this-togetherness' between senior decision-makers and staff were not, however, well received, particularly if they were perceived to go against rules imposed strictly on families:

> [Chief Executive] went to visit the adult unit the other day, when I was there, to see the staff that were redeployed. And I struggle a little bit – they taked [sic] an ITU nurse and a nurse from our unit had to show her round and I'm just like have they not got stuff that's better to do than show you around? And for me also, I think, crikey, our families, there's been a lot that has caused a lot of bad feeling. The families can't come in, but here the Chief Executive can wander round. It's like we had the Chief Nurse of [region] or something, come to our unit. And you're just like, I can't see my sister at the moment. Why, why on earth do I want to see you? Like, and I don't know if they feel that's morale boosting or something. But actually, it's just annoying. ... So it's really interesting what they maybe perceive boosts our morale to what actually does. And for me, people should not be wandering around units to visit who aren't necessary. I just think it's wrong. (Advanced nurse practitioner, paediatric intensive care)

Miscommunications, misunderstandings and a lack of transparency in decision-making, especially where stress levels were high, were experienced as problematic for relationships. This was particularly apparent in the early stages of the pandemic, where the coronavirus was not well understood, guidelines were changing rapidly, and staff members did not feel safe:

> And then obviously, you've got all of this protection that you think is protection, and then it changed quite quickly to no, you don't need to wear that anymore. And there was a lot of sort of conflict between teams, you know, Is this real? Are we sure? Is it because we don't have enough PPE [personal protective equipment]? Or is it you know, or is this true? (Advanced nurse practitioner, paediatric intensive care)

This emphasised the crucial importance of *transparent communication* in the maintenance of effective relationships between managers and healthcare professionals:

> [A]nd I think that initially [our management] were caught in this sort of difficult situation where they would, rather than say, we're not getting the PPE we need, or we want ... they would say, this is all you need. You don't need anything else. And so there's this sense of distrust and dishonesty that develops. (Paediatric intensive care consultant)

While the different priorities of management and patient-facing healthcare professionals were acknowledged ('so that is their ... priorities are different when it comes to management team' [neonatologist]), those with a clinical background often felt the burden of their organisational responsibilities: 'We're all really protective of our patients. Not everybody thinks that the good of the organisation some people quite rightly think of the good of their specialty. And it's, unfortunately my job to make the decision and say ... the balance of risk, it's you, that's the compromise' (Deputy Chief Nurse, Children's hospital).

These differing priorities introduced tensions into the relationships between individuals at different places in the hospital hierarchy, particularly where a healthcare professional was being asked to act in a way that they believed was contrary to the immediate needs of the patient, or family, in front of them:

> We begged the Trust to be able to let this woman in, she had two negative COVID tests ... And the trust wouldn't budge with letting her into the unit because she had to quarantine for two weeks. And the baby started deteriorating on day five, and gradually got worse. And I asked the Trust again to let her in. And they said no, because the baby wasn't for end of life care. So the only time that she'd be allowed in was if the baby died. And the baby did die on day seven. And that's the only time she saw her baby. ... You get annoyed with [management] and angry with them. And you think, you know, you just know you're following a government guideline. (Neonatologist)

In some circumstances this disjuncture between senior decision-makers and frontline healthcare professionals was experienced as very harmful, sometimes even to a healthcare professional's 'relationship' with who they were as a doctor, nurse or midwife:

> [A]nd you just didn't feel like you could help this family, you just felt like your hands are tied and you were restricted and that you couldn't deliver the level of care that you're used to being able to deliver. Which makes you feel rubbish about your job, and makes you feel rubbish going home. (Neonatologist)

For healthcare professionals based in the community, relationships with the patients or families they were visiting appeared to be less constrained by rules and policies:

> [A]nd it wasn't that there was midwives that were not sticking to the guidelines and the rules, they were just saying, actually on reflection, this lady probably does need a visit, or I'm not happy to leave her four weeks because you know, looking at the growth chart, or the blood pressure was just creeping up a little bit ... I wouldn't be happy to leave it. (Community midwife)

Community-based healthcare professionals (of whom the majority were midwives) described a more pragmatic, personal approach to patient care, in this case considering the general policy preference for remote 'visits':

> So I personally, would most definitely say if you're not happy with a phone call, if you feel like you need a visit, ... for you or the baby, you don't hesitate to contact us if you can't get me call the community office. So it's the way I personally practise. (Community midwife)

While healthcare professionals worried that different approaches might lead to inconsistencies in care, they recognised that everyone was aiming to offer the best care they could within the constraints imposed on them. Public participants across our focus groups explicitly situated good care in a supportive relationship with a particular healthcare professional who had gone the extra mile. Some healthcare professionals recognised the importance of such an approach too: 'the families always have my contact number for six months after discharge. And I always say to them, "You don't know where to go for advice, you don't know who to phone, phone me, and I will try and help"' (Specialist midwife).

Some healthcare professionals, both hospital- and community-based, felt more at risk than others and opted either to work from home or to decline community visits. This was sometimes experienced as burdensome by those who continued to work and to cover for shielding colleagues: 'people were very generous in allowing people to shield. ... Maybe a bit more challenging approach to is it correct that these people who maybe said they need to shield have to shield really?' (Consultant paediatric surgeon). However, relationships between team members generally facilitated the protection of colleagues who felt unable to carry out their usual role:

> I did pick up a few visits for a colleague who was just not happy to do that. And I absolutely understood that. Um yes, potentially, I was putting myself at risk, but I was using the correct PPE. And the visit needed to be done, the woman and baby needed to be seen. And actually, it wasn't right to say to my colleague, no that's your lady you need to do it. She didn't feel comfortable, and she didn't feel safe. And I absolutely understood that. (Community midwife)

The central theme across all the data was a recognition of the harm caused to *relationships* as a result of the changed working practices mandated by infection prevention and control measures:

> I think ... it's very hard to show empathy without somebody seeing your full face. So you have to work harder at the words that you use and building relationships ... because it's very difficult to, when you your whole face is covered up. ... You know, you're saying that you're very sorry that the baby's dying, and you've got like a ... a barrier between you. (Consultant neonatologist)

Relationships between healthcare professionals and patients were harmed:

> [Y]ou make people, women, less resilient during their pregnancy because we've harmed them or upset them. And then when it comes to being in labour, they're less resilient than they might otherwise be. And perhaps less trusting and, and then throw PPE on top of that, so you know, mask yourself up and glove yourself up and aprons and you introduce these barriers, you know, your midwife is not quite as friendly as she's in complete PPE even though she might be smiling behind her mask, it's harder to get close to someone. (Head of midwifery, DGH)

It was also noted that relationships between healthcare professionals and patients' families, and within the wider family networks of those who had suffered a bereavement were compromised:

> We had a child who died during the first lockdown, and she'd been with us, since she was about a week to two weeks of age. And so she hadn't met the family. So at the funeral, nobody knew this child, they didn't know her. And what mum was saying was that you are all the family, the nurses in intensive care and the nurses on the ward, you are my daughter's family, because you're the ones that have been there. And that was something that she even to this point now is really, really struggling [with] and gets angry, understandably. She's angry with most people ... but angry with us as a hospital, because we prevented family members actually coming in and seeing [her]. (Paediatric cardiac nurse)

The damage caused to relationships was often described as likely to have long-term consequences, both for families affected by difficult decisions, and for the healthcare professionals making them:

> [T]he impacts on those families, I think will last a lifetime. And we've done that. And the impact of losing a child lasts a lifetime anyway, but we managed to make it worse. ... I'll never forget it, I'll never forget those two examples. I'll never forget those. And we did that. And I was involved in it. And I feel I did a really bad job. (Neonatologist)

Frequently, the counterpoint to the distress experienced by healthcare professionals within the context of their patient relationships (including with patients' families) was the support available from colleagues:

> [W]hen you're tapping into your colleagues, you know, we were finding things out from each other, ... you know, when it was like, kind of sharing with each other new ways of working and how we'd found things that worked, and actually how we found this is really helpful. So, so we were supporting each other, and providing each other with the latest information. (Community midwife)

The nature of that collegial support was also significantly impacted by the requirements of social distancing and infection prevention measures: 'the support groups have all gone ... to Zoom they don't really work as well as having thirty to forty people in a room talking to each other about loss. ... We've just lost this element of support, ... and it's, it's hard' (Neonatologist).

Yet, the enduring availability of the relationships was valued. The availability of professional support from within the hospital was perceived positively: 'Our senior clinical managers are really, really great. So if they are aware that someone is struggling, they will absolutely provide whatever support is necessary' (Consultant neonatologist). Where it was made available to staff as well as patients, specialist support was valued: 'The Trust has employed psychologists in order to support staff sort of in the here and now and they are, you know, they are able to run workshops around resilience' (Head of Midwifery, DGH).

Our data clearly identified the central importance of relationships in healthcare, encompassing relationships between colleagues as well as between healthcare professionals and the patients and families in their care:

> We've just spent such a long time trying to ensure that parents are seen as equal partners and not visitors that they're part of our team and that the family, and the context of the family, is incredibly important when you're delivering care to a sick newborn baby or even a healthy newborn baby. (Consultant neonatologist)

Our findings thus make visible the harms to the enactment of healthcare relationships caused by practices and policies whose aim was to control the spread of the virus. While the virus was indirectly responsible, the regulations requiring social distancing and the consequent changes to 'usual' working practices were the direct cause of these harms, experienced particularly acutely in the (ideally) 'family-centred' maternity and paediatric services we were investigating. In the next section, we will situate these findings about the centrality of relationships in healthcare in a discussion of relational theories more broadly, drawing out their significance in the context of maternity and paediatric services.

Relationships recalibrated: theorising the stories we were told

Relational theorists have long suggested that it is in our 'networks of relationships' that we (our identities) are constituted (Nedelsky, 2011: 19; see Gilligan, 1977, 2014; Tronto, 1987; Barad, 2007). In suggesting this, they include widely drawn relationships that acknowledge the interdependence of humans and the natural world, less broadly drawn local societal relationships, and closer family relationships. Notions central to the idea that human beings are separate, bounded individuals are reconsidered and reimagined by reference to how we see ourselves in relation to other(s). Nedelsky (2011: 39), for example, argues that 'autonomy is made possible by constructive relationship (and undermined by destructive relationship)'. Similarly, it has been suggested that the concept of agency can be reframed so that it encompasses the capacity to 'affect and be affected' rather than (just) to understand and reflect (Deleuze and Guattari, 1987). In the discussion that follows, we review our findings through a relational lens, considering, in so doing, how a 'logic of relationality' (Lejano, 2021: 364) might form a better starting point than a logic of rationality for decision-making in the healthcare context.

Lejano (2021) offers the notion of a logic of relationality as a contrast to a conventional understanding of policy as underpinned by *rationality*, which he describes as prescription, guided by reason and knowledge, for pursuing desired ends, where the aim is to maximise the degree to which a decision conforms to a specified criterion. He suggests that a notion of relationality, where relationality describes the patterns and workings of relationships, better reflects how people work together in practice. Arguing that a rational, output-driven approach to rules and policies fails to attend to the way people work *within* relationships, he suggests that this explains the 'gap' that often develops in practice between the design of the rules, or policies, and the way they work or are interpreted by people whose work they are intended to direct.

The application of Lejano's relational logic would understand healthcare professionals, patients and their families not just as rule-setting and rule-following beings, but as *relational agents* whose interpersonal everyday interactions work out how the rules fit, and how policies are applied, to allow for a particular clinical set of circumstances, or attend to a particular patient's needs. Such a relational logic prioritises the sequences of actions and reactions that express and reinforce relationships. Viewed in this way, the rules are (to an extent) dynamic, creating an institutional approach which is negotiated to accommodate the various relational interactions and priorities.

An institutional approach underpinned by a relational logic, then, understands people within their networks (patients, healthcare professionals and families) as tending outwards, being constituted within and by their relationships, rather than existing as autonomous individuals in the Cartesian sense (Husserl, 1901). Similarly, Pollard (2015) has concluded that central tenets of relational ethics include (most importantly) mutual respect, engagement and responsibility. Gilligan (2014) has characterised relationality, feeling connected to other people and empathising with them, as an ethic of care and, developing this in the legal context, Herring (2013) has put forward four markers of care, situating the practice of caring specifically in a relational context, where care is an action, care meets a need, offers respect, and accepts responsibility.

Our research findings reconfirm the importance of these theoretical ideas in healthcare practice, highlighting the importance, for members of the public and for healthcare professionals, of emotional engagement, the meeting of needs (spiritual as well as clinical), mutual respect, and an enactment of responsibility for the wellbeing of patients, family members and colleagues. The caring relationships between healthcare professionals, their patients and the families of their patients, can, then, be understood as working to (co-)constitute their identities as *people-in-relationships*, as needs are met, responsibilities are accepted and both professional and personal selves are formed.

Attending in our analysis to the central importance of relationships in our data, we can theorise that the harms participants discussed were linked to the mandatory, non-negotiable nature of the infection prevention and control measures imposed during the pandemic. These strict measures, imposed (understandably, in the context of a public health emergency) to protect the ability of the system to continue to function, restricted (and in some cases removed) healthcare professionals' usual ability to negotiate or interpret policies and guidelines *with* their patients (and families) to fit the particular therapeutic context. Our suggestion is that we can make sense of our findings by reference to Lejano's (2021) logic of relationality. We posit that in what we might describe as 'usual' times,[7] hospital policy and decision-making sit within a combination of a logic of rationality (in terms of formulation of policy and guidance) *and* one of relationality when these policies and guidelines come to be interpreted and applied in practice.[8] In 'usual' times, the family is part of the team in maternity and paediatric services, and policies and guidelines are interpreted by the healthcare team *with* the patient and their family members, within the unfolding of a relationship embedded in an organisational context:

> But likewise, it's also really stressful with our parents who are very experienced, very involved in their children's care, for them to be excluded, because they really are part of our team. They are part of the treatment team for the child. Rather than just a supportive parent. Actually, it's really hard for staff to turn them away, because you know what it is that they're doing, and that they can. So I'd say probably that has been the greatest challenge for us. (Paediatric intensive care consultant)

Thus, the imposition of social distancing rules, visiting restrictions and the requirement to wear PPE, created largely *non*-negotiable barriers to relational engagement in the everyday practices our participants described. For the most part, the caring relationships *had* to give way. The consequent fracturing of the human interactions that our data describe sits at the heart of the ethical difficulties that were experienced by some of our interview participants and focus group discussants.

The case for a logic of relationality: the risks of disrupting relationships

The findings of our rapid review demonstrated that the safety of NHS staff was the most frequently occurring focus of guidance (Chiumento et al., 2021). This was also reflected in our interviews with senior managers.

> So ... the first thing that we thought about when we ... decided to restart our services was the safety of our staff, as we reintroduced face to face services. Then, of course, we also thought about safety of the families who were attending the hospital. ... So that was our overriding driver really, was how would we keep everybody safe ... how we would restart safely in a way that did not overcrowd our physical environment. And so we had a one parent or one carer per child rule. And we had risk assessments done on all the different physical spaces so that we knew how many people we could keep in those physical spaces. (Medical director, Foundation Trust)

In terms of organisational risk, then, healthcare professionals' safety seemed primarily to have been understood in terms of physical safety, particularly minimising exposure to COVID-19 in order to reduce as far as possible the impact of healthcare professionals' sickness. The (rational) aim of such a policy was the protection of the system as a whole, to ensure its ability to continue functioning (Chiumento et al., 2021).

> So there's a number of mutual aid things put in place that compromised our ability to restore our services within our traditional organisation, it became more of a system effort. But certainly staff availability, space and equipment and consumables were hard core factors and things that we have to work around. (Hospital Trust chief operating officer)

While this might seem appropriate as part of a pandemic response, we suggest that relational aims are (at least) equally as important, and should always feature in decision-making. For some senior decision-makers, it is clear that they did. Our data show that some managers were very aware of the negative impacts of rigid and inflexible infection prevention measures on healthcare professionals and patients, and of the resulting *ethical* challenges in terms of balancing infection prevention and supporting relationships:

> I mean, visiting is a big, big topic. And it was so upsetting for women and partners to miss out scans and some [to] miss birth and, you know, having to go home two hours after the birth and not being able to come to the ward. But it will also have to be done in a safe way. So there was lots of debate about, you know, is it safe to have, you know, how do we accommodate to safely – how do we take the view of staff into consideration? (Head of Midwifery, DGH)

This suggests that, whether in 'usual' times, during pandemics, or when the system is under pressure for other reasons, safety should be understood holistically, as encompassing not only physical health, but social, mental and moral health as well. Prioritising healthcare professionals' physical safety to the detriment of their mental and emotional wellbeing fails to recognise the longer term risks of burnout, or moral distress. While it is sad to note that 'absence, burnout and PTSD' are (now) recognised as significant strategic risks,[9] it is our contention that the risk of these harms could be mitigated with decision-making that recognises the moral significance of caring relationships to healthcare professionals, and the role such relationships can play in helping them negotiate ethical challenges.

The starting point for such a project, accepting that relationships are fundamental to healthcare, would be the development of organisational rules and policies that support, rather than stress, those relationships. This requires meaningful engagement with the ways in which relationships are enacted and valued, with a view to better understanding how to support them in practice. Starting with an analysis of the values that underpin the patterns and workings of relationships in healthcare, an ethical framework could be developed on and around which to base a discussion, involving stakeholders from across the hospital community, about supportive organisational rules and policies. While we accept that an ethical framework cannot (and should not) produce a recipe for decision-makers to follow, we suggest that a transparent ethical framework, co-constructed with relevant stakeholders (at the relevant time and in the relevant organisational context), offers a useful tool to support decision-making and help shape organisational practice. Drawing on our qualitative data and the ethical framework we developed inductively through our rapid review,[10] we set out in Table 2.1 the values we think are key, together with a suggestion of their meaning in the context of the caring relationships we have described above and how we suggest they might be incorporated into healthcare decision-making and policy-setting.[11]

Conclusion: arguing for an explicitly relational approach to healthcare policy and decision-making

It is our suggestion that, in foregrounding the importance of (the enactment of) caring relationships to the wellbeing of people across a hospital community, policy- and decision-makers will better engage and protect the people around whom the NHS is organised – members of the public, hospital staff, patients and their families. We do not argue that relationships are currently unrecognised in healthcare decision-making (this is clearly not the case), but, rather, that where rational outcomes (infection prevention and control, for example) are prioritised, this should be complemented by explicit

Table 2.1 Relationships and ethical values in healthcare decision-making

Ethical value(s)	What our data suggest this means in a healthcare setting	Recommendations for healthcare decision-making
Respect	The notion of respect encompasses enabling healthcare professionals to express their views and, where they do so, respecting their choices. Where this is not possible, transparency about *why* not is important.	Policies and procedures should support relationships, recognising what people need from others, what is (or has been) particularly difficult, and why, and with a view to making change where possible.
Balancing harms and benefits	Harms and benefits should be broadly conceived, encompassing physical, psychological, social, economic and ethical factors. Impediments to caring relationships may lead to moral harms.	Healthcare professionals' discretion in the interpretation of policies and procedures to support family (and other) relationships should be facilitated where possible.
Reciprocity	Reciprocity assumes a mutual exchange of benefit, or risk – and an assumption of responsibility. Within the context of the relationships we have considered, reciprocity is enacted, for example, in the tacit understanding that healthcare professionals will be kept safe at work, and that patients, healthcare professionals and other visitors to the hospital will adhere to infection prevention and control measures to help protect the wider hospital community.	Policies and procedures should be responsive to changes in the balance of benefits and risks, particularly where relationships are at stake. Reciprocity is at the heart of relationships, and an operationalisation of reciprocity in healthcare decision-making should, where possible, facilitate healthcare professionals' discretion to support (a) particular relationship(s) in a particular context.

Table 2.1 (Cont.)

Ethical value(s)	What our data suggest this means in a healthcare setting	Recommendations for healthcare decision-making
Fairness	A fair approach assumes that everyone matters equally, and that any disproportionate impact on one person (or a particular group) will be attended to appropriately. In the context of paediatric and maternity services, this would include thinking about the impact on future generations.	In the 'resetting' of NHS services, decision-making should be attentive to the interdependencies between healthcare professionals, patients and their families, and the importance of facilitating a fair application of policies and procedures in that context.
Accountability	Transparency, openness and information sharing are all aspects of accountability. In decision-making, or policy-setting (including, but not limited to, pandemic decision-making), transparency is crucial to underpin relationships founded on trust, in demonstrating how fairness and reciprocity are brought to bear, how harms are recognised and mitigated, and how respect is enacted.	Recognising the importance of transparency in relationships, decision-makers must develop and nurture an organisational culture of accountability. A culture of accountability would facilitate a softening or review of policy or procedure where required, by reference to a clear process to which all have access.

consideration of the impact on relationships. We found that this did happen in some settings, but that significant (moral) harm resulted in circumstances where it did not. In suggesting how attention might be paid to relationships, we return to Lejano's (2021) logic of relationality.

Lejano's central contention is that interpersonal relationships and everyday transactions are the mechanisms used to work policy into practice, so that policy is not experienced as 'prescription-and-implementation but as the workings of relationships' (2021: 361). Our data show that this policy 'dynamism' is a feature of healthcare professionals' normal negotiation of the rules in the context of their patient and professional relationships: respect for the patient's views, the provision of clear information to allow a transparent balancing of harms and benefits for that patient in that family, and attention to fairness in terms of the needs of other patients, are, we suggest, all features of 'usual' healthcare practice. The pandemic imported impediments to this dynamism in the shape of rules that were not amenable to negotiation. While, in our view, healthcare professionals and patients alike understood and accepted the necessity for this in the early acute phase of the pandemic, this changed during later waves of infection as understanding of the virus evolved. At this point, a focus on the impact of infection prevention measures on the *enactment of relationships* would have helped to inform decision-making. Returning to the story with which we opened this chapter, we suggest that the harms of refusing this new mother access to the ward where her sick baby was receiving care might have been mitigated by considering how a safe, fair and less harmful interpretation of the rules could be achieved. Our data suggest that the benefits of so doing would have been felt (in both the short and the longer term) not only by the young parents, but also by the healthcare professionals involved in caring for them and their dying baby.

It is, of course, much easier to suggest solutions in isolation, with the benefit of hindsight, and without having to account for the wider ripple effects of such negotiations on the wider community. For these reasons, this chapter is not intended simply to criticise the 'rational' approach to decision-making that characterised the approach to restoring non-COVID services in the 'reset' period that we were investigating. Rather, we suggest that the pandemic emergency offers an opportunity for reflection and learning, particularly in the context of a health service that, even in 'normal' times, is stretched. Our contention is that in setting policy, transparent and engaged communication that respects healthcare professionals' ability conscientiously and fairly to engage with others (colleagues, patients, family members and other carers) is crucial. By facilitating this, decision-makers can enable a greater harmony between policy, its application in action and the relationships within which all policy is embedded. Achieving such harmony will ensure that healthcare professionals, patients and their wider family and care networks are supported when critical, ethically difficult, decisions about the delivery of services are made, whether in pandemic times or otherwise.

Funding

The Reset Ethics research project was funded by the UK Research and Innovation Arts and Humanities Research Council, Grant number AH/V00820X/1.

Notes

1 Extract from a semi-structured interview with a neonatologist participating in the NHS Reset Ethics research project.
2 Such as, for example, the government's 'Guidance on pandemic flu', available at: www.gov.uk/guidance/pandemic-flu.
3 For a definition, and discussion, of moral distress, see McCarthy and Gastmans (2015).
4 A Maternity Voices Partnership (MVP) is an NHS working group: a team of women and their families, commissioners and providers (midwives and doctors) working together to review and contribute to the development of local maternity care. See MVP website, available at: https://nationalmaternityvoices.org.uk/.
5 The Healthwatch website is available at: www.healthwatch.co.uk/.
6 Quotations, taken from semi-structured interviews, are mostly reproduced verbatim but, on occasion, have been 'cleaned up' to aid readability.
7 Noting, as we do so, that the NHS experience over the course of a 'usual' year might also involve significant pressures on services at certain times, but that what we are taking to underpin our understanding of 'usual' is a public health context that does not require the imposition of any unusual or extraordinary measures.
8 Lejano (2021) notes that relational processes function along with rational/purposive rule systems in complementary fashion, and that we

should expect to find the relational to be operative everywhere, even in programmes that conform strictly to set rules and formal guidelines.
9 See, for example, Risk Register Report for the period to end August 2022 (as on 10 September 2022) for NHS University Hospitals Dorset Foundation Trust. Available at: www.uhd.nhs.uk/uploads/about/docs/bod/2022/6.3_risk_register_report.pdf.
10 This framework was developed from the Pandemic Flu Framework. See Chiumento et al (2021) for a description of the iterative development process.
11 In addition to the rapid review framework, we have also drawn on the 'team actions' set out in a document developed by one of our participating Trusts to guide decision-making on a paediatric ward.

References

Barad, K. (2007) *Meeting the Universe Halfway: Quantum Physics and the Entanglement of Matter and Meaning*, Durham, NC: Duke University Press.

Čartolovni, A. et al. (2021) 'Moral injury in healthcare professionals', *Nursing Ethics*, 28(5): 590–602.

Chiumento, A. et al. (2021) 'Which ethical values underpin England's National Health Service reset of paediatric and maternity services following COVID-19: a rapid review', *BMJ Open*, 11(6). http://dx.doi.org/10.1136/bmjopen-2021-049214

Deleuze, G. and Guattari, F. (1987) *A Thousand Plateaus: Capitalism and Schizophrenia* (trans. B. Massumi), Minneapolis: University of Minesota Press.

Gilligan, C. (1977) 'In a different voice: women's conception of the self and of morality', *Harvard Educational Review*, 47(4): 481.

Gilligan, C. (2014) 'Moral injury and the ethic of care: reframing the conversation about differences', *Journal of Social Philosophy*, 45(1): 89–106.

Herring, J. (2013) *Caring and the Law*, Oxford: Hart.

Husserl, E. (1901) *Logical Investigations* (trans. J. Finlay) vol. 2, London: Routledge.

Institute for Government (2022) 'Timeline of UK government coronavirus lockdowns and restrictions'. Available at: www.instituteforgovernment.org.uk/charts/uk-government-coronavirus-lockdowns (accessed 4 December 2023).

Jameton, A. (1984) *Nursing Practice the Ethical Issues*, Englewood Cliffs, NJ: Prentice-Hall.

Lejano, R. (2021) 'Relationality: an alternative framework for analysing policy', *Journal of Public Policy*, 41(2): 360–383. https://doi.org/10.1017/S0143814X20000057

McCarthy, J. and Gastmans, C. (2015) 'Moral distress: a review of the literature', *Nursing Ethics*, 22(1): 131–152.
Nedelsky, J. (2011) *Law's Relations: A Relational Theory of Self, Autonomy and Law*, Oxford: Oxford University Press.
Pollard, C. (2015) 'What is the right thing to do: use of a relational ethic framework to guide clinical decision-making', *International Journal of Caring Sciences*, 8(2): 362–368.
Stevens, S. and Pritchard, A. (2020) 'Second phase of NHS response to Covid-19'. Available at: www.england.nhs.uk/coronavirus/wp-content/uploads/sites/52/2020/04/second-phase-of-nhs-response-to-covid-19-letter-to-chief-execs-29-april-2020.pdf (accessed 4 December 2023).
Tronto, J. (1987) 'Beyond gender difference to a theory of care', *Signs: Journal of Women in Culture and Society*, 12(4): 644–663.

3

Evaluating post-pandemic plans for social care data infrastructures

Cian O'Donovan

Introduction: the lives data saves

'Suspected Covid' was the cause stated on Michael Gibson's death certificate. Mr Gibson died at the age of eighty-eight at the care home where he lived in Bicester, Oxfordshire, on 3 April 2020 after that care home took in a patient discharged from a hospital with coronavirus (COVID-19) (BBC News, 2022). Exactly four weeks later, Donald Harris, eighty-nine, died in Alton, Hampshire, after an outbreak of coronavirus in his care home (PA, 2022). The deaths of Gibson and Harris were preceded on 17 March by orders from central government to discharge from hospital more than twenty-four thousand older and clinically vulnerable people, many of whom ended up in care homes. Across these two months more than twenty thousand older people died of coronavirus-related causes in England. And through the pandemic's first wave, coronavirus was the greatest cause of death in care homes, and deaths in care homes occurred at greater frequency than in any other institutional setting (Dyer, 2022).

The pandemic exposed the long-standing neglect of care homes and wider social care infrastructure throughout the United Kingdom. In this chapter, I outline features of the data infrastructure that existed prior to the pandemic, scrutinising these features through three theoretic-analytic lenses: complexities within social care systems; the human values which shape what data measure and the decisions they inform; and the multiple scales at which data matter. I aim to show that a renewed infrastructure for producing and using social care data is urgently needed, not least because such data will play a useful role in evaluating the impacts of policy interventions, or indeed further neglect, across the sector. However, I also argue that with more data come further burdens on the people who collect it; tensions between those in the social care system who pay for data infrastructure and those who realise the value of the data; and sometimes difficult choices over how data come to categorise and value some individuals and groups, while neglecting others. My aim with this commentary is to offer insight into how improved social care data infrastructure might distribute these benefits and costs, and more importantly, be tuned to measure what matters most to people throughout our care systems.

Returning to the early days of the pandemic, how many care home deaths can be attributed to the mass discharge of elderly and clinically vulnerable people from hospital into care homes remains a matter of intense debate. But one thing has been resolved by the English High Court: the discharge decision itself was unlawful. In a case brought by the daughters of Michael Gibson and Donald Harris against the Secretary of State for Health and Social Care and Public Health England, presiding judges Lord Justice Bean and Mr Justice Garnham held that 'the drafters of the [discharge] documents of March 17 and April 2 simply failed to take into account the highly relevant consideration of the risk to elderly and vulnerable residents from asymptomatic transmission' (PA, 2022), concluding that this was 'not an example of a political judgment on a finely balanced issue' but a failure of decision-making (*Gardner & Harris v. Secretary of State for Health and Social Care*, 2022).

The judgment highlights at least two failures. The first is a failure of process. Lord Justice Bean and Mr Justice Garnham write: 'the decision to issue the April 2nd admission guidance in that form was irrational in that it failed to take into account the risk of asymptomatic transmission, and failed to make an assessment of the balance of risks' (Moore and Graham, 2022). Aggravating this failure of process was a long enduring failure across the English social care sector: a failure in the data infrastructures critical for keeping the health of social care service users under review, for regulating providers of social care services, and for holding to account decision-makers, planners and providers when things went wrong.

These failures are linked. In assessing the balance of risks for individuals, two things must be known at a population level: first, who, exactly, is at risk, and second, the degree to which that risk can be mediated, whether through action or by doing nothing. In practice, this arithmetic is complicated by a huge range of factors. For instance, comorbidities that vary across age, place, region and groups such as Black and Minority Ethnic people. Or the influence of environmental factors such as the quality of people's living conditions, whether in care homes, in sheltered housing or in their own homes (Apea et al., 2021; Katikireddi et al., 2021). However, even two years into the pandemic, no UK country could routinely identify care home residents, recipients of social care at home, care home workers or those providing care to people living at home (O'Donovan, Smallman and Wilson, 2021). Moreover, comprehensive data on the case mix and needs of residents was still absent. Simply put, even as the pandemic recedes, the government still does not know who is in care homes, where they are or what risks they face (Burton et al., 2022a). This is not only a failure of data: it is a failure of political and ethical responsibility too.

This chapter deals with two aspects of these data failures. First, I show that Michael Gibson, Donald Harris and other residents of UK care homes were *invisible* in national social care datasets, and I point to immediate causes and consequences of missing social care data during the pandemic. That is, missing data in terms of data that has not been created – it simply is not there, but also data that, colloquially, miss the point. For instance, routine health data that record clinical care may, in the context of care homes, neglect what matters most to residents themselves (Todd et al., 2020). Second, I use these stories to challenge already emerging narratives about pandemic data use. By the summer of 2021, a story of data's unalloyed successes in mitigating coronavirus was starting to be promoted by expert advocates of clinical data research. Pandemic rules that reduced information governance burdens and increased interlinkage between huge sets of data meant they could compile and analyse health research faster and at greater scale than ever, and their compelling story about data was one of lives saved (Department of Health and Social Care, 2021a; O'Donovan et al., 2021b). The real story is more complicated than that. Data, and the political and ethical decisions about who and what is datafied, is also implicated in jobs and lives that were made more vulnerable and stressful, and in lives that were lost.

The denominator problem in care home data

Accurate data and effective data infrastructures are critical for decision-making and planning at scale in representative democracies such as the United Kingdom. Data, and the scientific methods that underpin their production, allow politicians and civil servants to make decisions about citizens at a distance, and (should) enable those citizens to hold decision-makers to account when things go wrong (Ezrahi, 1990). But in March 2020, as UK leaders watched television reports full of death and fear in Italian hospitals, there was no reliable dataset they could query to inform life and death choices about whether to prioritise vulnerable people already occupying hospital beds in England, or to discharge them and make room for the thousands of COVID-19 patients predicted to flood National Health Service (NHS) wards. On 17 March the government did not understand who was in care homes, where those care homes were or for what duration of time people stayed in them (O'Donovan, Smallman and Wilson, 2021).

One major issue is what health system experts call a denominator problem, after the bottom number in a fraction (Lucas and Zwarenstein, 2015). This, in the care home context, is the number that represents the total population of people in care homes. Denominator problems often flow from issues of indicator construction, where indicators are categories of real things, such as beds or people, especially when estimated numbers are crude or out of date. Statisticians choose to count particular indicators in order to build models that facilitate regulation, prediction or control. Decisions about what indicator to choose often hinge on what can be counted easily (for instance, tallying beds is more straightforward than counting the wellbeing of the people occupying them), or what is being counted already. In the case of social care, for example, surveys instigated by the regulator might be used. Where secondary data sources are available, their use can be cheaper or quicker than gathering new data, but the downside is that secondary data often arrive stripped of the context for which they were originally produced.

Problems can arise in social care when indicators acting as static variables, again bed numbers are a good example, are incorrectly used to model dynamic population sizes and distributions of people *actually* moving – say patients moving between hospital and community care, or between jurisdictions. Over time, inaccuracies can lead to substantial measurement issues. When decision-makers do not know the denominator, they quickly end up with problems in basic calculations and false precision in the evaluation of services and, thus, the evidence base for policy.

These errors cost lives. When the denominator does not accurately represent the actual population of care home residents, reporting accurate segments of that population, or tracking homes that provide special kinds of care services, such as for residents over the age of eighty or with dementia, fair and useful allocation becomes impossible (Burton et al., 2020b). Even if we have a good sense of the care provided to the population overall, we have no idea about the care given to any one individual – or even a 'typical' individual.

The denominator problem exists because health and care infrastructures are not measuring all that really matters to residents, staff and care home operators. These problems are social as well as technical. For instance, the Capacity Tracker is an example of data infrastructure that was expanded rapidly during the early months of the pandemic in order to collect data about care home residents and make those data useful for decision-makers (NHS Vale of York Clinical Commissioning Group, 2021). The tracker was designed for efficiently allocating people being discharged from hospitals to care homes or other community care settings. One major problem was that the tracker counted stocks of beds and resources, but during a public health emergency what planners really need is information about risk and virus spread. For this, what is crucial is knowing the number of residents in each home, where they have come from and how healthy they are. However, the Capacity Tracker was intended to solve an *allocation* problem within a care sector constructed to function like a market. That's a necessary task, but one that is useful only in narrow terms.

The quality and comprehensiveness of care home data are made worse by other social and technological factors. The diverse settings of care homes make collecting standardised data difficult. Collection and maintenance of data are made more difficult still by poor digital infrastructures within many individual care homes. Regulatory incentives prioritise data gathering for monitoring *systems* and neglect data for evaluating impacts on *human residents*. And complex market arrangements and financial worries are disincentives for care home operators to share data within the sector, and between social care and NHS data systems. A major problem is that there are few trusted third-party data intermediaries who could increase trust in the sector and foster relationships between data providers based on common interests.

Why solving the denominator problem is important

The absence of these crucial data meant that adequate appraisal was impossible when it came to decisions about the March 2020 discharge. Further, the absence of sufficient data was of critical importance for ongoing planning during the pandemic. As is detailed elsewhere in this volume, gathering and sharing data became vital when decisions about allocation of personal protective equipment (PPE), enforcing action on care home staff and restricting visitors were being made, not least because care homes were housing and looking after residents who were typically older and less healthy than the general population, and so were more vulnerable to the most severe effects of coronavirus (Smallman et al., 2023). These points are of ongoing importance for anyone involved in operational and planning decisions in UK social care sectors.

This also matters because missing data contribute to a lack of public visibility and erode the ability of the individuals affected by such systematic underrepresentation to use the epistemic power of data to advocate for themselves in the public square. The lack of visibility for people in care flows from a lack of attention to, and resources for, the care sector – a fact that is not down to a single or specific institution but implicates a range of policies, institutions and practices over time. In short, the arrival of the coronavirus amplified existing inequalities of epistemic power, such that the power of data often benefited already well-represented groups while others were made ever less visible.

This continues to matter greatly because comprehensive data about the population that relies on well-functioning social care services like care homes remain patchy. Shockingly though, what we do know is that between March and July 2020, care home residents represented almost half of all coronavirus deaths and, by the end of December 2021, more than 26,935 residents of English care homes had contracted the virus and died (Curry and Oung, 2021).

These arguments are important, because together they make the case that the denominator problem is not just a technical issue to be solved by collecting ever more data in care homes or by instigating deeper surveillance of communities. Rather, these issues expose a wider problem across social care – that data come to categorise and value some individuals and groups while neglecting others. Moreover, these issues are not confined to care home data. Across social care, more denominator problems exist. People who pay for their own care, for instance, as well as adults in need of home care. In the first phase of the pandemic, more than 2,600 people with learning disabilities died in England, far in excess of deaths in the overall population (Kavanagh et al., 2021). Solving denominator problems across health and social care must be a priority for transformation agendas across the care sector.

Understanding care data infrastructures in context

Analysts of care home data know how to solve the denominator problem. Clinical data expert Dr Jenny Burton and colleagues have proposed seven technical and social interventions aimed at governments and health services (Burton et al., 2020a). These are:

1 providing reliable identification of care home residents and their tenure;
2 creating common identifiers to link data sources from different sectors;
3 creating individual-level, anonymised data that include mortality, irrespective of where death occurs;
4 investing in capacity for large-scale, anonymised linked data analysis within social care, working in partnership with academics;
5 recognising the need for collaborative working to use novel data sources, working to understand their meaning and ensure correct interpretation;
6 better integrating information governance rules and cultures to enable safe access for legitimate analyses from all relevant sectors;
7 creating a core national dataset for care homes, developed in collaboration with key stakeholders.

These solutions, or versions of them, have been discussed for years so what makes them so hard to implement? Three features of the social, physical and political environments in which care homes operate are worth considering here. These are the complexity of the social care system itself; the diverse norms of data infrastructures, and the values around which data infrastructures are built; and the different scales at which data are produced, used and made to matter.

Complexity

Care homes, like many other places in English society, are already data-rich environments, full of smartphones, smart meters, monitoring equipment and digital technologies. And yet systematically producing data that are useful to and usable by organisations such as local authorities has not been possible. To understand why, we need to consider the broader social care sector in which care homes operate. There is no single policy, funding or service stream that is widely understood as social care. Rather, social care is how society orders practices of care and distributes responsibilities and obligations for these practices between markets, the welfare state, voluntary sectors and communities and families (Daly and Lewis, 2000). The processes and practices that constitute social care thus take place across a hugely diverse and dynamic set of locations including, but not limited to, care homes. In the UK, care that is administered outside of hospitals and GP surgeries takes place in a patchwork of communities, small and medium enterprises, a small number of very large housing firms and charities – around nineteen thousand providers in all (The King's Fund, 2019). Approximately 1.6 million staff, managers, administrators and others are involved in delivering this care (Skills For Care, 2021). Responsibility for policy, legislation, standards and the allocation of funding is devolved to the four nations of the UK. The delivery of services is the responsibility of 152 local authorities in England, 22 in Wales, 32 in Scotland and 5 in Northern Ireland, each separately elected and responsible to their own local populations (Gray and Birrell, 2013).

In recent decades, this institutional and organisational complexity has served to obscure political neglect. Government policies since the turn of the century have created quasi-markets underpinned by ideologies of patient choice (Glendinning, 2016; Baxter et al., 2020). These politics and policies have failed (The Health Foundation, 2020; Allen and Tallack, 2021). They have resulted in the wide dispersal of key obligations, such as responsibility for funding care services and accountability when things go wrong, and the dilution of agency within the system to direct care to where it is needed most. By the time the pandemic hit in 2020, resources such as data, a skilled workforce and even beds were not there in the numbers required. In addition, funding was both insufficient and not getting through to where it was needed most (National Audit Office, 2018; Blakeley and Quilter-Pinner, 2019).

Data are especially important within this complex sector because decision-makers need information to resolve the significant issues that currently exist. They need to be able to identify problems in the social care system as a whole, and then come to an understanding of what would count as an improvement. The Adult Social Care Outcomes Framework (ASCOF) in England is a standardised collection of tools, rules, categories and data built for this purpose. Over the course of every year ASCOF aggregates data from a range of national and local surveys and databases, which is then used by central government for policy planning and monitoring, and by local authorities and councils with Adult Social Services Responsibilities (CASSRs) for measuring local performance and for benchmarking against other CASSRs (O'Donovan, 2022). However, people who are excluded from or unable to access local authority-funded care services are invisible in ASCOF data. Thus the annual reports produced using ASCOF data do not contain information that accurately reflects the quality of life of people receiving and delivering care (Jones and Meyer, 2021) and, crucially during the pandemic, data with which to assess and hold accountable, in close to real time, the delivery of care, the state of organisations providing care, and decision-makers directing resources.

System complexity is further increased by the constantly changing and dynamic nature of the system itself and what experts call system performativity (Wilson, 2021). Performativity is important because interventions in the present can and will impact the future of the system, and it is the evolving framing or shaping of the system itself that can influence these changes. System designers know this, and frameworks such as ASCOF are designed, at least in part, to performatively drive behaviour across multiple levels of governance. Scholarship on improving accountability in social care notes the importance of good mechanism design within frameworks such as ASCOF to protect against unintended consequences (Naylor, 2018).

The principal role care infrastructure plays in people's lives changed rapidly during the peak of the pandemic. At the time, the top priorities for many staff were minimising virus transmission, infections and deaths. Capacity Tracker data designed to allocate beds were now being used to make decisions about distributing PPE. With the provision (or lack) of equipment, staff were adapting their work practices to new realities on the ground. At the same time, policymakers learned more about the risks posed to residents by the virus and came under increasing scrutiny for their delayed response to coronavirus in care homes. In response, government legislated to require all care home staff to receive a vaccination (Department of Health and Social Care, 2021b). Discussing the efficacy and ethics of vaccine mandates are beyond the scope of this chapter, save that the controversy highlights important ethical implications for data infrastructure: for any data system or set of indicators, however carefully constructed, what counts as a breach of a duty of care or a violation of privacy is not something that can be described once and for all. Rather, what constitutes a violation is partly constituted by individual expectations and sectoral norms, which will themselves change in response to external crises and government action. Taking performativity in systems seriously means rethinking the assumption that there is a static ethical reality, which can accurately be mapped and modelled with ethical concepts and theories. Thus, system design needs also to be attentive to the potential for values to change with circumstances.

Values

Data play an important role in clarifying the relationship between an idealised concept of how care in homes should be delivered and the lived realities of people's lives as measured by specific variables. In doing this, data are imprinted with the value judgements of those choosing what data to collect, and those giving consent for that collection. These value judgements are not universal. What is valued in data can and often does differ significantly across health and social care settings. For instance, values guiding data collection and interpretation in hospitals often differ from those prioritised in care homes. Moreover, individual care homes are themselves complex settings, within which a vast milieu of human values, interests and normative concerns combine.

So, what values matter within social care data infrastructures and where can we find these? First, ideas and values about how care *should* be delivered and measured do not form separately from understandings already present in policy debates, within local authorities and on the ground which are often institutionalised as rules, regulatory frameworks and best practices. For instance, ASCOF (Measure 1L) reports 'the proportion of people who use services or carers who reported that they had as much social contact as they would like' and this is recorded via the annual Adult Social Care Survey (NHS Digital, 2021). Indicators in surveys like these typically stage individuals and their rights as service users as the ethical unit of analysis. This staging is, itself, a design choice that has implications for how care is assessed and delivered in society.

In addition to the hundreds of value judgements made during the construction of individual measures and indicators, there are overarching logics driving data design and use. One major issue is the focus by local authorities commissioning services on measures of *time and task* (a measure of resource efficiency) rather than on individual or community outcomes, which are much more difficult and costly to count. Also, the survey methods used to produce data tend to discount people who fund their own services and are not recorded in local authority figures. Is this because these people are not deemed important enough to be datafied, or do they subsequently become unimportant because they are missing from data? Whatever the rationale, the implications are significant. Because of the quasi-market organisation of care services, accountability is structured through consumer choice. Thus, excluding segments of the population from data effectively excludes their voices from governance in the sector completely.

Of course, care itself is also a value; one that directs attention to neglected things and devalued doings (Puig de la Bellacasa, 2011) such as the hidden labours of care workers (Lutz, 2013), or the marginalised groups being excluded from social services. Recognising the value and potential of care in this way, socially and relationally as well as economically, depends on a different understanding of what care actually is: not as a bundle of market-based services but as a set of relationships that depends on human connection (Cottam, 2021). Relational values of care are notable in their commitment to egalitarian practices and the affording of agency to those receiving care (Arora et al., 2020). This means that processes for measuring and directing care should extend beyond counting resources and indicators of services and, in so doing, usefully report on the heterogeneous relationships that make up caring practices. Yet, insofar as these relations and aspects of everyday lives are captured at all by existing measures and methods in data infrastructures, it seems system designers have not thought them worth knowing.

Even in this brief discussion, then, it is clear that there are tensions between decentralised logics of how data encode what matters to people and groups on the ground; market-oriented logics of accountability and governance across the sector; and imperatives for centralised command and control logics that might allow the government take a firm grip in public health crises such as coronavirus.

Multiple scales

These tensions between conflicting values can be mapped across the different scales at which data infrastructures operate. For instance, in the early days of the pandemic, decisions about health and care were rapidly centralised within government departments and at the level of national administrations. Thus, a critical part of assessing data infrastructure is understanding and addressing the conflicts and tensions that come from putting data to use across different scales.

Our assessment of these ethics and politics is guided by Melanie Smallman (2022) who offers a set of questions that heuristically guide our investigation. These include, for instance, questions that address tensions between comprehensive coverage of populations and over-surveillance of groups and communities. As discussed above, the initial production of care home data usually focuses on the level of individuals, through the work of care home staff or residents filling out surveys. During the pandemic, many staff members worried about the increased data collection responsibilities imposed by the Capacity Tracker. As well as increasing the burdens on staff members, this amplified existing problems of low pay and time scarcity (Jones and Meyer, 2021; O'Donovan, 2021b) and is an example of the tensions that can exist between local, institutional and system-level demands – in this case, the benefits for local authority and central decision-makers of collecting care home data versus the burdens on the care staff.

At the individual scale, there are also important questions of who benefits and who is burdened by data. For instance, what kind of accountability processes are in place to ensure that rights to privacy surrendered by individuals are duly matched by gains from increased pandemic surveillance. Similar questions arise at the scale of groups and communities. We know that existing social, economic and health inequalities were made much worse by the pandemic and contributed to unequal outcomes, including higher death rates, among people from Black, Asian and Minority Ethnic communities compared with the general population (Health and Social Care, and Science and Technology Committees, 2021). We also know that increased exposure to COVID-19 as a result of people's housing and working conditions played a significant role in unequal outcomes for people working in health and care jobs (Health and Social Care, and Science and Technology Committees, 2021). Data that fail to convey the heightened risks at these group and community scales to the level of national decision-making further exacerbate racist and unequal structures across care sectors.

Time also matters. As the crisis stage of the pandemic ends in the UK, a comprehensive review of the temporary pandemic data measures is now in order. Measures brought in during crises have a way of becoming permanent and of being applied in situations beyond those used to justify them. Infrastructures lock in routines and practices which, once established, can be difficult to alter. For instance, obligations on care staff to collect data as part of the Capacity Tracker programme is one such issue. Another issue is concerns around data governance arrangements that have reduced information governance burdens to allow researchers and planners to more quickly access and analyse population health data (O'Donovan, 2021a). Researchers will be reluctant to let these measures go. But this stance risks overlooking dramatic shifts in public attitudes around how data are collected and used, driven by huge overspends on NHS Test and Trace, ongoing scandals relating to the procurement of PPE and the opaque nature of deals with large technology firms for enterprise data systems (Bharti et al., 2021). Given that timescales of pandemics are rarely certain at the start, it is critical, then, that as the crisis evolves into something else, data infrastructures and the manner in which they shape organisational, institutional and social arrangements across a range of scales are revisited and reassessed.

Policy for social care data

So, what can an approach that foregrounds complexity, values and multiple scales tell us about the prospects for emerging responses and long-term plans that aim to transform data use in social care? What is most curious about transformation policies and reports is that already the pandemic response has been hailed as a victory for accelerating data use in health and care, and for scaling up data infrastructures that support these uses. Take Data Saves Lives, the UK government's first major consultative study on data use in health and social care during the pandemic (Department of Health and Social Care, 2021a). The consultation's title neatly foreshadowed its findings, focusing in the main on how health data played a significant role in decision-making and planning associated with mitigating and adapting to the virus (Department of Health and Social Care, 2022b).

The Goldacre Report, a parallel consultation sponsored by the Department of Health and Social Care, intensified a focus on large-scale digital research infrastructure and the imposition of flexible information governance regimes that accelerated clinical research on the virus (Goldacre, 2022). These reports praised pandemic changes in data governance, and the practices and infrastructures that supported rapid data use in health and social care sectors. But they contained little discussion about the complexity of social care, the unintended consequences of increased data gathering in care homes, or the impact of data beyond clinical research, for instance, how data shapes and obscures who is made accountable in the sector.

Data Saves Lives and the Goldacre Report are important because they form the rhetorical and evidentiary basis of subsequent White Papers, strategic plans and policy proposals for addressing long-term neglect in English social care. For instance, the 2021 Social Care White Paper (Department of Health and Social Care, 2021c) recognises that transformation in the sector is urgently needed and, specifically, that this must include improving data infrastructures. But, in relying so much on Data Saves Lives and the Goldacre Report, the 2021 White Paper replicates their neglect of certain people, places and issues. The White Paper also advances and anticipates commitments relating to a series of subsequent consultations.[1] Across these strategies, there are at least three significant proposals for digital transformation in social care. The first proposal is renewed attention to evolving and improving the ASCOF, including efforts to link health and care records across organisations and institutions. This is to be welcomed, at least to the degree to which this project will embed and make explicit the diverse ways in which social care services, service users and outcomes can be measured and ultimately valued by government and society.

The second proposal revolves around the integration of a wide variety of services, procurement and operational strategy at a local, place-based level. The creation of Integrated Care Systems within the Health and Care Act 2022 (UK Government, 2022) has led to a major reorganisation and convergence of NHS systems and services in the first instance with the integration of social care often a secondary concern. Cresswell, Sheikh and Williams (2022) identify three key issues with convergence: a lack of clarity on exactly what systems are to converge and at what scale; open questions about how to conceptualise convergence and concerns that more important than identifying single systems for interconnection is a job of aligning cultures and practices of care across complex settings; and the need to develop a sense of shared direction towards a future state – questions about how future integrated systems will be maintained and evolved remain open.

Ignoring these issues risks reinforcing concerns about top-down management. Indeed, a worry reported in informal conversations among social care staff and decision-makers is that the NHS will continue to take precedence in the allocation of resources, marginalising or alienating social care services and users (O'Donovan, 2021b). As far as data use is concerned, the technical job of linking data between organisations and institutions must, in my view, be preceded by an ethical analysis of the reasons for, and the terms on which, data are used in different settings and at different scales. It is not sufficient to consider the political, personal and ethical implications during design and build phases of data infrastructure. Procedures that ensure ongoing accountability for residents, staff and informal carers are critical for good governance.

The third proposal is concerned with accelerating the construction of digital research infrastructure such as the trusted research environments (TREs) championed in the Goldacre Report (Goldacre, 2022). TREs are technical platforms and standardised data practices designed to enable access to sensitive data for authorised projects and researchers only, thereby minimising risk of data release or exposure. Social care data analysts are making use of TREs, especially in work that makes use of interlinked healthcare data (Burton et al., 2019, 2022b). But, given the relative immaturity of social care data infrastructure compared with those of hospital and GP patient data, advocates of health data research are likely to steer the agenda for investment in TREs in the immediate term.

Conclusions: what social care data need to measure

So, what is missing from forward plans and policy? First, policies might better recognise heterogeneity in social care systems, in term of individuals, groups, organisations and the institutional players with a stake in the sector. Planners must acknowledge that different groups will benefit from data differently and, given the drive towards further interconnection and convergence, the assumptions on which plans are based must be spelled out. The benefits of data cannot be taken to be the same in different parts of the social care system. Plans must, then, clearly distinguish between how different groups in society interact with health and social care data, and experience data-informed decisions. Finally, the attention to TREs is a welcome step in acknowledging that public perception of data infrastructure matters, but the issue of building public trust in the wider health and social care system, while at the same time broadening data use, cannot be addressed through technical specifications alone.

Problems with data about care homes often result from choices in design, or from neglect. In both cases, these things offer opportunities for redesigning the system, and maintaining it differently (and better). At the level of individual care homes, for instance, it will be important to consider how to design and implement a data-informed, data consent system that is appropriate for a cohort of people who are not digital natives. Approaching these challenges from a systemic perspective, the key question is not so much how best to measure the system on a static snapshot basis (the how many beds approach), but rather requires a strategic analysis. This is a bigger-picture question of how to structure institutions, networks, incentives and accountabilities in ways that maintain and strengthen how the system distributes obligations such as care and accountability over time (Wilson, 2021). And given that there is no universal and enduring measure of what we mean by *care* in care homes, it is, in my view, better to adopt a pluralist approach. This means acknowledging that the problems revealed by data are historical, contextual and differ from place to place and, further, that solving one problem may often contribute to worsening others. Because of these factors, different kinds of data, and the expertise to gather and use those data, are required.

The greatest challenges in UK social care today are tackling cost pressures and demographic needs, ensuring people currently excluded from services get the help they need, building staff capabilities, and improving the quality of services and outcomes for users. These challenges are urgent and have been for years. Improving data infrastructures is a pre-condition to the design and operationalisation of post-pandemic strategies that aim to tackle these issues and evaluate their impacts. Failure to do so risks making things worse.

But perhaps, too, there exists an opportunity for a more radical agenda for data in social care. Backed by a series of White Papers in 2021 and 2022, the English government again promised major reform of the social care sector (Department of Health and Social Care, 2021c), but by April 2023 a major roll-back was under way as hundreds of millions of pounds of funding for workforce training and housing adaptation was postponed (Bottery, 2023). The most useful progress towards meeting the challenges that this chapter describes, then, might not start with the data. Rather, the first step should be to ensure that social care cultivates the kind of political capital across society as well as within the sector that makes breaking these promises impossible. This is a fundamental prerequisite to ensuring that staff who work with data in care homes and across the social care sector are empowered to lead satisfying work lives, on terms that align with best practice and shared values. Recognising the value of social care, and of the relations of care that underpin the sector, will afford both staff and people who depend on social care status and respect in society and within the infrastructures through which we know them in data.

Funding

The chapter was supported by the UKRI-funded UK Pandemic Ethics Accelerator, Data Use workstream, grant number AH/V013947/1 and UKRI-funded Environmental impacts of digital services for health and wellbeing in the home, grant number EP/V042130/1.

Note

1 Consultations and strategies reviewed for this chapter include 'Health and social care integration: joining up care for people, places and populations' (Department of Health and Social Care, 2022c), and the 2022 Cavendish Report (Cavendish, 2022) as well as a specific digital strategy for health and social care (Department of Health and Social Care, 2022a) which in turn builds on the 2021 Adults Social Care Technology and Digital Skills Review (Blake et al., 2021).

References

Allen, L. and Tallack, C. (2021) 'Sunak was silent on social care when action is needed now', *The Health Foundation*, 10 March. Available at: www.health.org.uk/news-and-comment/blogs/sunak-was-silent-on-social-care-when-action-is-needed-now (accessed 18 March 2021).

Apea, V. J. et al. (2021) 'Ethnicity and outcomes in patients hospitalised with COVID-19 infection in East London: an observational cohort study', *BMJ Open*, 11(1): e042140. https://doi.org/10.1136/bmjopen-2020-042140

Arora, S. et al. (2020) 'Control, care, and conviviality in the politics of technology for sustainability', *Sustainability: Science, Practice, and Policy*, 16(1): 247–262. https://doi.org/10/gh65np

Baxter, K., Heavey, E. and Birks, Y. (2020) 'Choice and control in social care: experiences of older self-funders in England', *Social Policy and Administration*, 54(3): 460–474. https://doi.org/10/gh63t2

BBC News (2022) 'Covid: discharging untested patients to care homes "unlawful"', *BBC News*, 27 April. Available at: www.bbc.com/news/uk-england-61227709 (accessed 5 April 2023).

Bharti, N. et al. (2021) 'Public trust, deliberative engagement and health data projects: beyond legal provisions', *Engaging Science, Technology, and Society*, 7(1): 125–133.

Blake, M. et al. (2021) *NHSX Adult Social Care Technology and Digital Skills Review*. NHSX. Available at: www.ipsos.com/en-uk/nhsx-reviews-published-digital-technology-innovation-and-digital-skills-adult-social-care (accessed 6 June 2022).

Blakeley, G. and Quilter-Pinner, H. (2019) *Who Cares? The Financialisation of Adult Social Care*. London: Institute for Public Policy Research. Available at: www.ippr.org/research/publications/financialisation-in-social-care

Bottery, S. (2023) 'Reform of adult social care: vanishing over the horizon', *The King's Fund*. Available at: www.kingsfund.org.uk/blog/2023/04/reform-adult-social-care-vanishing-over-horizon (accessed 14 April 2023).

Burton, J. K. et al. (2019) 'Identifying care-home residents in routine healthcare datasets: a diagnostic test accuracy study of five methods', *Age and Ageing*, 48(1): 114–121. https://doi.org/10.1093/ageing/afy137

Burton, J. K. et al. (2020a) 'Closing the UK care home data gap: methodological challenges and solutions', *International Journal of Population Data Science*, 5(4). https://doi.org/10/gjhqcf

Burton, J. K. et al. (2020b) 'Evolution and effects of COVID-19 outbreaks in care homes: a population analysis in 189 care homes in one geographical region of the UK', *The Lancet Healthy Longevity*, 1(1): e21–e31. https://doi.org/10.1101/2020.07.09.20149583

Burton, J. K. et al. (2022a) 'Developing a minimum data set for older adult care homes in the UK: exploring the concept and defining early core principles', *The Lancet Healthy Longevity*, 3(3): e186–e193. https://doi.org/10.1016/S2666-7568(22)00010-1

Burton, J. K. et al. (2022) 'Understanding Pathways into Care homes using Data (UnPiCD study): a retrospective cohort study using national linked health and social care data', *Age and Ageing*, 51(12): afac304. https://doi.org/10.1093/ageing/afac304

Cavendish, C. (2022) 'Social care reform: an independent review by Baroness Cavendish', GOV.UK. Available at: www.gov.uk/government/publications/social-care-reform-an-independent-review-by-baroness-cavendish (accessed 6 January 2023).

Cresswell, K., Sheikh, A. and Williams, R. (2022) '"Managed convergence" in health system digitalisation', *Journal of the Royal Society of Medicine*, 115(8): 284–285.

Curry, N. and Oung, C. (2021) 'Fractured and forgotten? The social care provider market in England', Nuffield Trust. Available at: www.nuffieldtrust.org.uk/research/fractured-and-forgotten-the-social-care-provider-market-in-england (accessed 7 May 2021).

Daly, M. and Lewis, J. (2000) 'The concept of social care and the analysis of contemporary welfare states', *The British Journal of Sociology*, 51(2): 281–298. https://doi.org/10/cgvrr4

Department of Health and Social Care (2021a) 'Data saves lives: reshaping health and social care with data (draft)', GOV.UK. Available at: www.gov.uk/government/publications/data-saves-lives-reshaping-health-and-social-care-with-data-draft/data-saves-lives-reshaping-health-and-social-care-with-data-draft (accessed 5 July 2021).

Department of Health and Social Care (2021b) 'Everyone working in care homes to be fully vaccinated under new law to protect residents', GOV.UK. Available at: www.gov.uk/government/news/everyone-working-in-care-homes-to-be-fully-vaccinated-under-new-law-to-protect-residents (accessed 15 May 2023).

Department of Health and Social Care (2021c) 'People at the heart of care: adult social care reform', White Paper, London: HM Government. Available at: www.gov.uk/government/publications/people-at-the-heart-of-care-adult-social-care-reform-white-paper (accessed 1 June 2022).

Department of Health and Social Care (2022a) 'A plan for digital health and social care', HM Government. Available at: www.gov.uk/government/publications/a-plan-for-digital-health-and-social-care/a-plan-for-digital-health-and-social-care (accessed 29 June 2022).

Department of Health and Social Care (2022b) 'Data saves lives: reshaping health and social care with data', London: HM Government. Available at: www.gov.uk/government/publications/data-saves-lives-reshaping-health-and-social-care-with-data/data-saves-lives-reshaping-health-and-social-care-with-data (accessed 29 June 2022).

Department of Health and Social Care (2022c) 'Health and social care integration: joining up care for people, places and populations', HM Government. Available at: www.gov.uk/government/publications/health-and-social-care-integration-joining-up-care-for-people-places-and-populations/health-and-social-care-integration-joining-up-care-for-people-places-and-populations (accessed 3 July 2022).

Dyer, C. (2022) 'Covid-19: policy to discharge vulnerable patients to care homes was irrational, say judges', *BMJ*, 377: o1098. https://doi.org/10.1136/bmj.o1098

Ezrahi, Y. (1990) *The Descent of Icarus: Science and the Transformation of Contemporary Democracy*, Cambridge, MA: Harvard University Press.

Gardner & Harris v. Secretary of State for Health and Social Care (2022). Available at: www.judiciary.uk/judgments/gardner-harris-v-secretary-of-state-for-health-and-social-care/ (accessed 5 April 2023).

Glendinning, C. (2016) 'Long-term care and austerity in the UK: a growing crisis', in B. Greve (ed.) *Long-term Care for the Elderly in Europe: Development and Prospects*, Abingdon: Routledge, 107–125. https://doi.org/10.4324/9781315592947

Goldacre, B. (2022) 'Better, broader, safer: using health data for research and analysis', London: Department of Health and Social Care. Available at: www.gov.uk/government/publications/better-broader-safer-using-health-data-for-research-and-analysis/better-broader-safer-using-health-data-for-research-and-analysis (accessed 8 April 2022).

Gray, A. M. and Birrell, D. (2013) *Transforming Adult Social Care: Contemporary Policy and Practice*, Bristol: The Policy Press.

Health and Social Care, and Science and Technology Committees (2021) 'Coronavirus: lessons learned to date', Sixth Report of the Health and Social Care Committee and Third Report of the Science and Technology Committee of Session 2021–22, HC-92, House of Commons. Available at: https://committees.parliament.uk/publications/7496/documents/78687/default/ (accessed 12 October 2021).

Jones, L. and Meyer, J. (2021) 'Suddenly social care data matters! So let's future proof it properly', *DACHA Study*, 7 July. Available at: https://dachastudy.com/suddenly-social-care-data-matters-so-lets-future-proof-it-properly/ (accessed 20 October 2021).

Katikireddi, S. V. et al. (2021) 'Unequal impact of the COVID-19 crisis on minority ethnic groups: a framework for understanding and addressing inequalities', *Journal of Epidemiology and Community Health*, 75(10): 970–974. https://doi.org/10.1136/jech-2020-216061

Kavanagh, A. et al. (2021) 'Improving health care for disabled people in COVID-19 and beyond: lessons from Australia and England', *Disability and Health Journal*, 14(2): 101050. https://doi.org/10/gkf7ct

Lucas, H. and Zwarenstein, M. (eds) (2015) *A Practical Guide to Implementation Research on Health Systems*, Brighton: Institute of Development Studies.

Lutz, P. A. (2013) 'Surfacing moves: spatial-timings of senior home care', *Social Analysis*, 57(1): 80–94. https://doi.org/10/f3rpck

Moore, V. L. and Graham, L. D. (2022) '*R (Gardner and Harris) v Secretary of State for Health and Social Care and Others [2022] EWHC 967*: scant regard for Covid-19 risk to care homes', *Medical Law Review*, 30(4): 734–743. https://doi.org/10.1093/medlaw/fwac044

National Audit Office (2018) 'Adult social care at a glance', London: National Audit Office.

Naylor, A. (2018) 'Facilitating care insight to develop caring economies', Future Care Capital. Available at: https://futurecarecapital.org.uk/research/facilitating-care-insight-to-develop-caring-economies/ (accessed 9 December 2023).

NHS Digital (2021) 'Measures from the Adult Social Care Outcomes Framework', *NHS Digital*. Available at: https://digital.nhs.uk/data-and-information/publications/statistical/adult-social-care-outcomes-framework-ascof (accessed 29 July 2021).

NHS Vale of York Clinical Commissioning Group (2021) 'Capacity tracker'. Available at: www.valeofyorkccg.nhs.uk/about-us/partners-in-care-1/care-home-and-domiciliary-care-staff-area1/capacity-tracker/ (accessed 14 May 2021).

O'Donovan, C. (2021a) 'Debate needed on post-pandemic rules for medical data', *Research Professional News*, 1 December. Available at: www.researchprofessionalnews.com/rr-news-political-science-blog-2021-12-debate-needed-on-post-pandemic-rules-for-medical-data/ (accessed 6 December 2021).

O'Donovan, C. (2021b) 'Issues and options for UK social care data policy: a report from the LCTcovid.org webinar What policy for UK social care data needs to do now', University of Oxford: UK Pandemic Ethics Accelerator. Available at: https://ukpandemicethics.org/wp-content/uploads/2021/11/Data-use-EA-LTCcovid-seminar-report-16-November.pdf (accessed 6 December 2021).

O'Donovan, C. (2022) 'Accountability and neglect in UK social care innovation', *International Journal of Care and Caring*, 7(1): 67–90. https://doi.org/10.1332/239788221X16613769194393

O'Donovan, C., Smallman, M. and Wilson, J. (2021a) 'Making older people visible: solving the denominator problem in care home data', University of Oxford: UK Pandemic Ethics Accelerator. Available at: https://ukpandemicethics.org/library/making-older-people-visible-solving-the-denominator-problem-in-care-home-data/ (accessed 11 June 2021).

O'Donovan, C. et al. (2021b) 'Consultation on the Data Saves Lives strategy: written evidence submitted by the UK Pandemic Ethics Accelerator's Data-Use workstream', University of Oxford: UK Pandemic Ethics Accelerator. Available at: https://ukpandemicethics.org/wp-content/uploads/2021/07/Data-Saves-Lives-submission-from-the-UK-Pandemic-Ethics-Accelerator-Date-use-workstream.pdf (accessed 23 July 2021).

PA (2022) 'Women whose fathers died from Covid win High Court challenge against Government', *The Independent*, 27 April. Available at: www.independent.co.uk/news/uk/crime/government-high-court-matt-hancock-covid-health-secretary-b2066472.html (accessed 5 April 2023).

Puig de la Bellacasa, M. (2011) 'Matters of care in technoscience: assembling neglected things', *Social Studies of Science*, 41(1): 85–106. https://doi.org/10/fsm9c4

Skills for Care (2021) 'The state of the adult social care sector and workforce in England', Skills for Care Workforce Intelligence. Available at: www.skillsforcare.org.uk/adult-social-care-workforce-data/Workforce-intelligence/publications/national-information/The-state-of-the-adult-social-care-sector-and-workforce-in-England.aspx (accessed 3 January 2022).

Slaughter, A.-M. and Cottam, H. (2021) 'We need a new economic category', *The Atlantic*, 23 September. Available at: www.theatlantic.com/ideas/archive/2021/09/new-economy-caregiving/620160/ (accessed 6 October 2021).

Smallman, M. (2022) 'Multi scale ethics: why we need to consider the ethics of AI in healthcare at different scales', *Science and Engineering Ethics*, 28, article 63. https://doi.org/10.1007/s11948-022-00396-z

Smallman, M. et al. (2023) 'Data ethics in an emergency', in C. Redhead and M. Smallman (eds) *Governance, Democracy and Ethics in Crisis-decision making: The Pandemic and Beyond*. Volume IV. Manchester: Manchester University Press.

The Health Foundation (2020) 'Five key insights on COVID-19 and adult social care', Newsletter feature, 30 July. Available at: www.health.org.uk/news-and-comment/newsletter-features/five-key-insights-on-covid-19-and-adult-social-care (accessed 18 March 2021).

The King's Fund (2019) 'Key facts and figures about adult social care', London: The King's Fund. Available at: www.kingsfund.org.uk/audio-video/key-facts-figures-adult-social-care

Todd, O. M. et al. (2020) 'New horizons in the use of routine data for ageing research', *Age and Ageing*, 49(5): 716–722. https://doi.org/10/gjhqck

UK Government (2022) *Health and Care Act 2022*. Available at: www.legislation.gov.uk/ukpga/2022/31/contents/enacted (accessed 16 May 2023).

Wilson, J. (2021) *Philosophy for Public Health and Public Policy: Beyond the Neglectful State*. Oxford; New York: Oxford University Press.

4

Data ethics in an emergency

*Melanie Smallman, Cian O'Donovan,
James Wilson and Jack Hume*

Over the past five or more years, as the power of data-driven technologies has become increasingly apparent, the field of data ethics has emerged as an interdisciplinary field, drawing upon important ideas from bioethics, particularly around the rights of the individual. Notwithstanding the plurality of ethical guidelines, prior to the coronavirus (COVID-19) pandemic, reviews of guidelines for ethical AI and data technologies have described a strong convergence around five key ethical principles: transparency; justice and fairness; non-maleficence; responsibility and accountability; and privacy (Jobin et al., 2019; Fjeld et al., 2020; Hagendorff, 2020).

The pandemic has, however, seen data used in new and accelerated ways, and in a very different context. The urgent need to find public health measures to reduce the spread of the disease and to develop new vaccines and new treatments has been coupled with the promise that more data can help (Wood et al., 2019; Davalbhakta et al., 2020). In the UK in particular, this increased collection and use of data – specifically via the initially planned NHS contact tracing app – raised serious concerns about users' privacy, as the app would have gathered and stored anonymised data from the app on a central NHS database. The Ethics Advisory Group to NHSX on the COVID-19 Contact Tracing App put forward a series of ethical issues to be considered in the development of the app, highlighting the importance of value, impact, security and privacy, accountability, transparency and control in securing public trust (Ethics Advisory Group, 2020).[1]

However, for some scholars, the increased possibility for surveillance of citizens afforded by these apps pushed ethical concerns further, raising issues about human rights and privacy (Sekalala et al., 2020a, 2020b), while others have argued that there is a danger that heightened levels of surveillance become more publicly acceptable (Couch et al., 2020) in a context in which capacity for critical scrutiny is disarmed (Philip and Cherian, 2020).

In medical and research ethics, there have been important discussions about the appropriateness or sufficiency of traditional research ethics in the context of a pandemic. Research ethics aims to protect research participants from any unacceptable risks presented by new treatments or the research process as set out in the WMA (World Medical Association) Declaration of Helsinki – Ethical Principles for Medical Research Involving Human Subjects, 1964 (WMA, 1964). A life-threatening pandemic raises new questions about what risks should count as 'unacceptable': a prominent example was the performance of Challenge Trials, in which participants were deliberately infected with COVID-19 (Killingley et al., 2022). Arguably, the widespread presence of a novel infectious disease calls for lower levels of risk aversion towards untested treatments as we try to expand our arsenal of medical defence against a new disease (Edwards, 2013). In recognition of that, and the pressures that pandemics put upon researchers, in 2016 the World Health Organization (WHO) released specific Guidance for Managing Ethical Issues in Infectious Disease – a set of guidelines for conducting ethical research during a pandemic (World Health Organization, 2016). These guidelines acknowledge that 'during an infectious disease outbreak there is a moral obligation to learn as much as possible as quickly as possible, in order to inform the ongoing public health response, and to allow for proper scientific evaluation of new interventions being tested'.

In this chapter, we argue that we need a similar debate and set of guidelines for ethical data use in an emergency such as a pandemic. By examining how data have been used during COVID-19 in the UK, we reflect on the value of the ethical principles that currently govern the ethical use of data and consider whether they have been sufficient during the pandemic.

COVID-19 and data in the UK

To begin reviewing the effects of data on the pandemic we examined third-party timelines of policy decisions relating to the pandemic in England – for instance, the Institute of Government

Timeline and supporting data (Institute for Government, 2021). We aimed to identify key 'moments' where data played prominent or particular roles. This flagged up three 'data episodes' which we investigated further and briefly describe below. These 'data episodes' were selected to help us understand the different ways that data were involved and used in the pandemic, rather than to give an historical account of the pandemic. We have described the time period in which these episodes were situated for contextual purposes, but it is important to note that these are not necessarily discrete events. The timescale in which these episodes (and their effects) occurred are complex, intertwining and far reaching – factors that generate many important, and perhaps novel, ethical considerations.

Episode 1: the data pandemic (March 2020)

On 16 March 2020, the then British Prime Minister Boris Johnson began a series of daily press conferences to update people on the COVID-19 pandemic. In his very first press conference, he explained that 'our objective is to delay and flatten the peak of the epidemic by bringing forward the right measures at the right time, so that we minimise suffering and save lives' and that 'it looks as though we're now approaching the fast growth part of the upward curve' (UK Government, 2020c).

Four days later, on 20 March 2021, more than 600 public health, epidemiology and medical experts sent a letter to the government arguing that data, models and experience elsewhere were clearly pointing to a need for urgent measures to stop the spread of COVID-19 (Iacobucci, 2020). Infographics of the model produced by Imperial College, showing the predicted exponential growth of COVID-19 cases with and without lockdown measures, spread across social media. On 23 March 2021, Boris Johnson announced the first UK-wide lockdown, which would come into force a few days later on 26 March 2021. Dramatically restricting people's movement and social contact, the Prime Minister explained that the purpose of this lockdown was to protect the NHS. 'To put it simply, if too many people become seriously unwell at one time, the NHS will be unable to handle it – meaning more people are likely to die, not just from Coronavirus but from other illnesses as well'

(UK Government, 2020b). From the very start, this was a data pandemic, with graphs, infographics and figures driving public concern and, in turn, government action.

Reinforcing this, in March 2020, a team from the digital arm of the NHS (NHSX) were assembled and tasked with developing a contact tracing app. The app 'appeared to be at the very centre of the government's strategy to beat coronavirus and help us all emerge from lockdown' (Cellan-Jones, 2020). Using mobile phones' Bluetooth functionality, the app would keep a record of any other users that the phone came into contact with, sending an alert and instruction to quarantine if a close contact tested positive. Importantly, this NHS app would have gathered and stored anonymised data on a central NHS database. Even before the app was tested in the Isle of Wight in May 2020, concerns about data security and privacy were prevalent. In June 2020, plans to develop the NHS's own app were dropped in favour of one based on technology provided by Google and Apple – ostensibly because this technology was more reliable, although this version of the app also had the privacy benefit of not passing data onto a single official database (Wise, 2020). During the first year after its launch, the app was used regularly by approximately 16.5 million users (28 per cent of the total population), sending approximately 1.7 million exposure notifications. The privacy-preserving features of the app made measuring its effects difficult, but Wymant et al. (2021) estimate that, between 24 September 2020 and the end of December 2020, it reduced case numbers in England and Wales by between 108,000 and 914,000.

Alongside these new forms of data collection, existing regulations and guidance on the use of confidential patient information were relaxed on a temporary basis. Under the Health Service (Control of Patient Information) Regulations 2002 (COPI), a COPI notice was sent to a wide range of NHS bodies on 20 February 2020, requiring them to process and make available confidential information to support the COVID-19 response. This had the effect of setting aside the common law duty of confidentiality where data was processed by health professionals for COVID-19 purposes during the time that the COPI notices remained in force (they expired on 30 June 2022).

The COPI notices provided the legal basis for the setting up of the NHS COVID Data Store, in March 2020, which brought 'together multiple data sources from across the health and care system in England into a single, secure location'. Creating such a centralised NHS data store 'would have taken years under normal circumstances', but under the COPI notices, 'the data store was established at pace, while protecting the privacy of our citizens' (NHS Transformation Directorate, undated). The US tech company, Palantir, known for its work on behalf of the CIA, played a key role in the setting up and running of the backend for the data store. Palantir initially contracted to work for a fee of £1, with its contract being extended for four months in June 2020 for a further £1 million. This contract was extended again, in December 2020, for another two years, this time for £23 million, without the contract at any stage undergoing a formal tendering process (Downey, 2020).

Adding to the data involved in the government's response to the pandemic, in mid-April 2020, the UK's Office of National Statistics (ONS) working with the University of Oxford, IQVIA, Lighthouse Laboratory at Glasgow, UKHSA, the University of Manchester and the Wellcome Trust, piloted a coronavirus (COVID-19) infection survey, inviting 20,000 people in England to provide a blood and swab sample at regular intervals. In August 2020, this sample size was expanded and from October 2020 extended to the whole of the UK, such that by the spring of 2022, the survey was collecting and analysing 120,000 blood samples every month. As well as being used to estimate the rate of transmission of the infection, the survey provided sociodemographic information about those contracting COVID-19.

Episode 2: care homes scandal (May 2020)

By 15 May 2020, press conferences from 10 Downing Street featuring politicians and senior government science advisers had become a daily feature of pandemic life. That day, the Secretary of State for Health and Social Care – standing in for the Prime Minister and announcing a new support package for the social care sector – assured the public that a 'protective ring' had been placed around UK care homes (Merrick, 2021). He was responding to concerns that the government's stated priority to protect the NHS had resulted in neglect elsewhere across other public sectors – specifically in social care.

In particular, in March 2020, thousands of older people had been discharged from hospital, many ending up in care homes without having been tested for COVID-19. Gathering and sharing data became vital when decisions about allocation of PPE, enforcing action on care home staff and restricting visitors were being made, not least because care homes were housing and looking after residents who were typically older and less healthy than the general population, and so were more vulnerable to the most severe effects of COVID-19. Yet basic data about who lived in which care home were missing. This is perhaps unsurprising given that while care homes are information- and data-rich environments, it was also a sector experiencing decades of neglect, underfunding and being undervalued. In addition, different stakeholders and different care homes had different information requirements. But this absence of data created fresh vulnerabilities (and effectively rendered invisible) an already extremely vulnerable population. In the first wave, COVID-19 was the greatest cause of death in care homes, and deaths in care homes occurred at greater frequency than in any other institutional setting (Dyer, 2022). However, because of insufficient testing at the time and an absence of data about who was in which care home, it is likely that the exact figures of COVID-19-related infections and deaths – and whether Hancock's 'protective ring' had been effective – will never be known.

Since then, some social care data infrastructure has improved. The ONS began to report (on an experimental basis) the numbers of self-funded people in care homes on 15 October 2021; and the Capacity Tracker, which was used by administrators to locate available care home beds, was adapted to monitor levels of infection, PPE and, ultimately, vaccination nationally. Nevertheless, even by the summer of 2022, no UK country was able routinely to identify who was resident in care homes, who was receiving social care at home or who was working in or visiting a care home or the home of someone receiving care in the community (O'Donovan et al., 2021; Burton et al., 2022). Moreover, comprehensive data on the case mix and needs of residents are still absent. Simply put, even as the pandemic recedes, the government does not know who is in care homes, where they are or what risks they face.

Episode 3: It ain't over 'til it's over: the end of the pandemic? (February 2021–22)

In February 2021, as the COVID-19 vaccine rollout was reaching the majority of the UK population and the Prime Minister faced mounting pressure from his own party to ease restrictions, the Westminster government stated in its 'Roadmap out of lockdown' (22 February 2021) that the government would be 'guided by data, not dates'. Shortly afterwards, the UK saw the arrival of the delta and the omicron variants of the virus, which, although they were significantly more transmissible and caused infection rates to escalate, in combination with the effectiveness of the vaccine, ultimately caused a lower proportion of deaths than the initial strain.

The soaring number of cases that came with the initial relaxation of lockdown measures in the summer of 2021 resulted in what became known as the 'pingdemic', when more than 500,000 alerts and instructions to self-isolate were sent out via the contact tracing app in the week ending 7 July 2021. Coming at a time when the seven-day rolling death rate was under 30 per day,[2] the disruption being caused led many individuals to delete the app.

The government launched a 'Living with COVID-19' plan on 21 February 2022. This involved a phased reduction or elimination of various COVID measures, including dropping asymptomatic testing in schools (on 21 February 2022); removing the requirement for routine contact tracing and self-isolation after a positive test result (on 24 February 2022); removing powers from local authorities to process data under the COPI regulations (which lapsed on 1 July 2022); and removing free testing (asymptomatic and symptomatic) for the general public (on 1 April 2022) (see Mehlmann-Wicks, 2022; GOV.UK, 2022).

With the end of free testing, of the test and trace system and of the legal duty to report cases of COVID-19, the most significant source of data about the spread and levels of COVID-19 infections was effectively disrupted, and the official government COVID data reports[3] moved from daily, to weekly updates on 1 July 2022.

The COPI regulations also lapsed on 1 July 2022. Nevertheless, COVID cases continued to rise, with more than 200,000 new cases reported on 24 March 2022,[4] and deaths within 28 days of positive test remained high, averaging over 200 per day for much of April 2022.

Concurrent with relaxation of COVID regulations, one of the biggest scandals in British politics ('Partygate') was unfolding. Between December 2021 and January 2022, allegations emerged that the Prime Minister and staff at Downing Street had broken the government's own COVID rules by holding a series of parties during lockdown. In December 2021, civil servant Sue Gray was tasked with investigating these allegations, after the Cabinet Secretary, the Prime Minister's initial choice to lead the inquiry, had to recuse himself when one of the parties was revealed to have occurred in his private office. Public outrage about the allegations coincided, in January 2022, with the growing concern among right wing Conservative MPs about the number of restrictions on freedoms still being imposed through the COVID-19 regulations, and a number of Conservative backbenchers began to call for Boris Johnson's resignation. On 25 January 2022, the Metropolitan Police also announced a criminal investigation into Downing Street parties. On 13 April 2022, Boris Johnson and his wife Carrie were served with fixed penalty notices for breaking lockdown rules, with Johnson eventually being forced to resign as Conservative Party leader on 7 July 2022.

Insights

These three 'data episodes' raise a number of questions about whether the values standardly discussed in data ethics are sufficient to guide us in a pandemic.

Ethics advice in an emergency and the risk of 'ethics washing'

At a practical level, the standardly discussed data ethics values have been adopted in the UK government's Data Ethics Framework (UK Government, 2020a), which specifically highlights the values of transparency, accountability and fairness. But neither this framework, nor the principles developed specifically by the ethics advisory board for the NHS COVID-19 app, nor the government's Pandemic Influenza Ethical framework, appear to have been made use of in government decision-making during the pandemic (Gadd, 2020). It was therefore unclear whether, and which, ethical considerations were given weight within government decision-making.

This is problematic in the first instance because, in the UK, there are clear rules to ensure those in public life are acting in the public interest, enshrined in the 'Nolan Principles of Public Life': Selflessness, Integrity, Objectivity, Accountability, Openness, Honesty and Leadership. The lack of transparency about if and how ethical frameworks were used would arguably have fallen short of the Openness and Accountability called for by the Nolan Principles, and the Good Decision-making principle of the 'Pandemic Influenza Ethical Framework'.

Beyond that, however, there is also a risk that the logic of ethics advice could uphold the logic that produces the unethical effects, by providing the possibility of ethical cover and compliance. Taking ethical advice could thus be a way to give the impression that actions are ethically justifiable. While we argue that a framework for data ethics in an emergency is needed, being able to evaluate whether and how such frameworks and sources of ethics advice are used is important too.

Time, scale, data infrastructure and democracy

Measures that might appear appropriate during a pandemic may become problematic if they are incorporated into everyday life – perhaps, as some have argued, risking gently moving us towards a less democratic and more authoritarian state (Cooper and Aitchison, 2020; Thomson and Ip, 2020). Furthermore, the impact on particular groups that have already been well described elsewhere (for instance, Hendl et al., 2020) are likely to be compounded by the persistence of COVID surveillance infrastructure. Considering questions of time and persistence seems to be vital – but seemingly absent in the pandemic response – when looking at infrastructures that affect large numbers of people and institutions, such as discussions around the test and trace system and the contact tracing app (discussed in Episode 1 above).

Arguably, existing ethical frameworks could incorporate these elements. For instance, time in the form of intergenerational fairness would seem to be a reasonable consideration within the 'fairness' agenda. But, in the absence of a structured way of ensuring time and scale are factored into ethical considerations, the point at which the trade-off between privacy and public health becomes less favourable for the majority of the public becomes difficult to identify. As a result, the data infrastructure put in place and the data collected during COVID-19 risk taking on a permanence. For example, while the COPI notices lapsed at the end of June 2022, the appetite for large-scale health data infrastructure built by commercial companies persisted. In April 2022, NHS England announced a £240 million contract for a Federated Data Platform for the NHS, the value of which was upgraded to £360 million in July 2022.

Scheuerman (2006) has written about the problem of ending emergency powers in relation to the additional powers acquired by the US President in the aftermath of 9/11. He argues that the distinction between ordinary and emergency law easily becomes blurred, while the mechanisms for containing emergency powers are unclear. Scheuerman advocates for legal processes to constrain and potentially end any emergency powers (for instance requiring increasing super-majorities in parliament to support extensions of temporary powers). Here, we add that these questions should also be built into ethical evaluations of data collection and use.

Role of data/absence of data in creating vulnerabilities

As we have described, concerns about privacy and over-surveillance appear to have been at the fore of ethical discussions and frameworks relating to COVID, and the contact tracing app in particular. However, the care homes episode shows very clearly that the opposite (*under*-surveillance) could present a risk too – an issue that was neglected in ethical considerations.

This danger presented itself on two fronts: first, as an ongoing absence of data about the health, wellbeing and whereabouts of residents and staff in care homes; second, as an absence of appropriate data sharing and linkage between care home providers, the care sector more broadly and other public domains which relied upon such data to make decisions and to evaluate the impact of those decisions in real, or close to real, time.

Sustained absences in these data were especially pernicious in social care, as they fed into decisions about the distribution of resources, responsibilities and obligations between markets, the welfare state, voluntary sectors and families. Without these data, decisions about who is deemed to require or deserve care, about how resources such as PPE should be distributed and how the effectiveness of decisions can be monitored and measured, were very difficult, if not impossible.

A renewed data ethics for pandemics that is attentive to these issues would trace how data systems simultaneously tackle and sustain diverse vulnerabilities, while at the same time reflexively addressing unintended systemic impacts.

Role of data in co-producing authority to act

Looking at all three data episodes, it becomes apparent that data played a role in providing the authority to act: First, at the start of the pandemic, the Prime Minister drew upon figures and statistics based on the data to build a picture of the pandemic as a growing threat that required him to introduce stringent measures to limit people's personal freedoms. For instance, his daily press conferences typically opened with a series of slides showing graphs and figures, which journalists and the public were invited to query and share. We argue that at the start of the pandemic, given the serious restrictions that needed to be imposed by a Conservative leader who was politically disposed to increase, not limit, freedoms, data provided additional legitimacy to act, beyond that provided by political arrangements at the time. The authority and legitimacy to act were co-produced through the sense of objectivity that data offered, along with the political powers of the office of prime minister.

Second, during the care-home episode, the absence of data was implicated in the neglect of care home residents; without the data to back up the need to act, residents, family members and staff on the ground had little by way of authority to redirect centralised resource distribution to care homes, or to engage in democratic challenges to the story emerging at government level of a 'protective ring' having been constructed around the sector.

Others have previously described the power of numbers and how data and political arrangements co-produce power and legitimacy (for instance Ezrahi, 1990; Porter, 1996). Looking at the third episode (the end of the pandemic), we argue that it was the complex and co-productive relationship between data, politics, authority and legitimacy, and a prime minister under threat and needing to consolidate power, that played the key role in creating the sense that the pandemic was over in the UK. For most Britons, the COVID-19 pandemic ended in the spring of 2022, when restrictions were lifted and test and trace stopped. Yet, in June 2022, the *British Medical Journal* warned that one in fifty people in the UK tested positive that week (Wise, 2022). Even in the well-vaccinated UK, the pandemic was far from over. Despite claims to 'follow the data not dates', we argue that when the Prime Minister's authority was challenged after the 'Partygate' scandal, he wrested back power by tipping the balance of the co-productive relationship towards his *political* authority by ending the collection and publication of key *data* – most notably the daily numbers of new infections. In the absence of these data, the authority and legitimacy to act – and therefore decision-making power – was produced by the position of prime minister alone.

Conclusions

In this chapter we have identified and described three key 'episodes' in the COVID-19 pandemic where data played a key role – and raised significant ethical issues. In so doing, we have shown that during the pandemic, emergency measures were intimately linked with the collection and analysis of data at an accelerated pace. Data, therefore, formed a key part of the logic by which power was wielded over the public. Moreover, the authority given by the seeming objectivity of data was sufficiently powerful to enable the British Prime Minister and government to enact, and then repeal (arguably too quickly), severe restrictions on civil liberties in the UK.

We have drawn attention to the range of consequences this has had for our lives as citizens. Some of these consequences are acutely ethical: increased surveillance capability; invisibility and neglect; placement of power and political authority to act; and the potential to 'ethics wash', yet typically escape the scrutiny of 'traditional' data ethics frameworks. We therefore conclude that a set of ethical guidelines for the use of data in an emergency needs to be developed to help improve the use of data in future pandemics.

In particular, these emergency data ethics need to take account of how the sense of objectivity, and therefore the authority to act, are co-produced by data and political arrangements; the effect of data gaps in creating vulnerabilities; a mechanism for structuring ethics thinking to look at the timescale of the pandemic and to consider the conditions under which the emergency will have ended and when normal regulations should once again apply. This last point is not inconsiderable given that, in the UK at least, data and the sense of the pandemic were intertwined, with the end of the pandemic being produced by the end of data collection and reporting, rather than the end in infections.

Finally, any emergency ethics framework needs concrete principles and clear ways of evaluating and accounting for their uptake, since, as we have shown, ethics frameworks may prove ineffectual if they are too abstract and indeterminate, allowing multiple plausible interpretations and accommodations. For instance, the issues we have raised here, such as the long-term effects of data collection, could be accommodated within ideas around privacy and security, but appear not to have been. More concrete principles and ways of evaluating their uptake seems necessary in the face of creeping powers and surveillance during a pandemic.

In saying this, we are not denying that data – and indeed emergency powers – can play a legitimate role in achieving public safety during a pandemic. But we argue that emergency contexts set different standards for data ethics and government transparency, because emergencies give rise to uncomfortable decisions about whose wellbeing ought to be prioritised and how. Neither the 'trust-based' reasons for transparency, common to some public health discourse, nor the 'rights-based' approach taken by traditional data ethics, may be sufficient in the context of a pandemic to ensure that a desirable balance is struck between health benefits, erosions of privacy and costs to democracy.

Funding

The chapter was supported by the UK Pandemic Ethics Accelerator, Data Use workstream, grant number AH/V013947/1.

Notes

1 This ethics advisory board was disbanded when the UK government made the decision to move from an NHS developed app to one based on Google/Apple technology.
2 Deduced by comparing the deaths data here: coronavirus.data.gov.uk/details/deaths?areaType=nation&areaName=England with the COVID-19 app dataset at stats.app.covid19.nhs.uk/. Available at: stats.app.covid19.nhs.uk/data/covid19_app_country_specific_dataset.csv?cacheBuster=1660125249358
3 coronavirus.data.gov.uk/
4 Infection rates reported here: systems.jhu.edu/research/public-health/ncov/

References

Burton, J. K. et al. (2022) 'Developing a minimum data set for older adult care homes in the UK: exploring the concept and defining early core principles', *The Lancet Healthy Longevity*, 3(3): e186–e193.

Cellan-Jones, R. (2020) 'Coronavirus: what went wrong with the UK's contact tracing app?' *BBC News*, 20 June. Available at: www.bbc.com/news/technology-53114251 (accessed 16 August 2022).

Cooper, L. and Aitchison, G. (2020) 'The dangers ahead: COVID-19, authoritarianism and democracy', London School of Economics. Available at: eprints.lse.ac.uk/105103/4/dangers_ahead.pdf (accessed 16 August 2022).

Couch, D. L., Robinson, P. and Komesaroff, P. A. (2020) 'COVID-19: extending Surveillance and the panopticon', *Journal of Bioethical Inquiry*, 17(4): 809–814. https://doi.org/10.1007/s11673-020-10036-5

Davalbhakta, S. et al. (2020) 'A systematic review of smartphone applications available for corona virus disease 2019 (COVID19) and the assessment of their quality using the Mobile Application Rating Scale (MARS)', *Journal of Medical Systems*, 44(9): 164. https://doi.org/10.1007/s10916-020-01633-3

Downey, A. (2020) 'Palantir awarded £23m deal to continue work on NHS COVID-19 data store', *Digital Health* (blog), 21 December 2020. Available at: www.digitalhealth.net/2020/12/palantir-awarded-23m-deal-to-continue-work-on-nhs-covid-19-data-store/ (accessed 16 August 2022).

Dyer, C. (2022) 'COVID-19: policy to discharge vulnerable patients to care homes was irrational, say judges', *BMJ*, 377: o1098. https://doi.org/10.1136/bmj.o1098

Edwards, S. J. L. (2013) 'Ethics of clinical science in a public health emergency: drug discovery at the bedside', *The American Journal of Bioethics*, 13(9): 3–14. https://doi.org/10.1080/15265161.2013.813597

Ethics Advisory Group (2020) 'Report on the work of the Ethics Advisory Group to NHSX on the COVID-19 contact tracing app'. Available at: covid19.nhs.uk/pdf/ethic-advisory-group-report.pdf (accessed 16 August 2022).

Ezrahi, Y. (1990) *The Descent of Icarus: Science and the Transformation of Contemporary Democracy*, Cambridge, MA: Harvard University Press.

Fjeld, J. et al. (2020) 'Principled artificial intelligence: mapping consensus in ethical and rights-based approaches to principles for AI', Berkman Klein Center Research Publication No. 2020-1, Cambridge, MA: Harvard University.

Gadd, E. (2020) 'Is the government using its own ethical framework?' The Nuffield Council on Bioethics, 24 April. Available at: www.nuffieldbioethics.org/blog/is-the-government-using-its-own-ethical-framework?fbclid=IwAR15mGREtJMO4ktXsk_wO0J9c3q3tXcBSyAjSZOvcAphFL2-kkd07q-3RAI (accessed 16 August 2022).

GOV.UK (2022) 'PM Statement on Living with COVID: 21 February 2022'. Available at: www.gov.uk/government/speeches/pm-statement-on-living-with-covid-21-february-2022 (accessed 29 April 2022).

Hagendorff, T. (2020) 'The ethics of AI ethics: an evaluation of guidelines', *Minds and Machines*, 30: 99–120. https://doi.org/10.1007/s11023-020-09517-8

Hendl, T., Chung, R. and Wild, V. (2020) 'Pandemic surveillance and racialized subpopulations: mitigating vulnerabilities in COVID-19 apps', *Journal of Bioethical Inquiry*, 17(4): 829–834. https://doi.org/10.1007/s11673-020-10034-7

Iacobucci, G. (2020) 'COVID-19: UK lockdown is "crucial" to saving lives, say doctors and scientists', *BMJ*, 24 March. Available at: www.bmj.com/content/368/bmj.m1204 (accessed 16 August 2022).

Institute for Government (2021) 'Timeline of UK Government coronavirus lockdowns and restrictions', The Institute for Government, 9 April. Available at: www.instituteforgovernment.org.uk/charts/uk-government-coronavirus-lockdowns (accessed 16 August 2022).

Jobin, A., Ienca, M. and Vayena, E. (2019) 'The global landscape of AI ethics guidelines', *Nature Machine Intelligence*, 1(9): 389–399. https://doi.org/10.1038/s42256-019-0088-2

Killingley, B. et al. (2022) 'Safety, tolerability and viral kinetics during SARS-CoV-2 human challenge in young adults', *Nature Medicine*, 28: 1031–1041. https://doi.org/10.1038/s41591-022-01780-9

Mehlmann-Wicks, J. (2022) 'BMA briefing: living with COVID-19 response', BMA, 24 May. Available at: www.bma.org.uk/advice-and-support/covid-19/what-the-bma-is-doing/bma-briefing-living-with-covid-19-response (accessed 16 August 2022).

Merrick, R. (2021) 'Matt Hancock denies making "protective ring around care homes" claim, despite saying it live on TV', *The Independent*. Available at: www.independent.co.uk/news/uk/politics/matt-hancock-care-homes-protect-claim-b1860484.html (accessed 16 August 2022).

O'Donovan, C., Smallman, M. and Wilson, J. (2021) 'Making older people visible: solving the denominator problem in care home data', UK Pandemic Ethics Accelerator. Available at: ukpandemicethics.org/library/making-older-people-visible-solving-the-denominator-problem-in-care-home-data/ (accessed 16 August 2022).

Philip, J. and Cherian, V. (2020) 'The psychology of human behavior during a pandemic', *Indian Journal of Psychological Medicine*, 42(4): 402–403. https://doi.org/10.1177/0253717620935574

Porter, T. M. (1996) *Trust in Numbers: The Pursuit of Objectivity in Science and Public Life* (reprint edition), Princeton, NJ: Princeton University Press.

Scheuerman, W. E. (2006) 'The powers of war and peace: the Constitution and foreign affairs after 9/11', *Perspectives on Politics*, 4(3): 605–607. https://doi.org/10.1017/S1537592706530361

Sekalala, S. et al. (2020a) 'Analyzing the human rights impact of increased digital public health surveillance during the COVID-19 crisis', *Health and Human Rights*, 22(2): 7–20.

Sekalala, S. et al. (2020b) 'Health and human rights are inextricably linked in the COVID-19 response', *BMJ Global Health*, 5(9): e003359. https://doi.org/10.1136/bmjgh-2020-003359

NHS Transformation Directorate (undated) 'The NHS COVID-19 data store: putting data at the centre of decision making'. Available at: transform.england.nhs.uk/key-tools-and-info/data-saves-lives/improving-health-and-care-services-for-everyone/the-nhs-covid-19-data-store-putting-data-at-the-centre-of-decision-making/ (accessed 16 August 2022).

Thomson, S. and Ip, E. C. (2020) 'COVID-19 emergency measures and the impending authoritarian pandemic', *Journal of Law and the Biosciences*, 7(1): lsaa064. https://doi.org/10.1093/jlb/lsaa064

UK Government (2020a). 'Data ethics framework'. Available at: www.gov.uk/government/publications/data-ethics-framework (accessed 16 August 2022).

UK Government (2020b) 'Prime Minister's statement on coronavirus (COVID-19): 23 March 2020', GOV.UK. Available at: www.gov.uk/government/speeches/pm-address-to-the-nation-on-coronavirus-23-march-2020 (accessed 16 August 2022).

UK Government (2020c) 'Prime Minister's statement on coronavirus (COVID-19): 16 March 2020', GOV.UK. Available at: www.gov.uk/government/speeches/pm-statement-on-coronavirus-16-march-2020 (accessed 16 August 2022).

Wise, J. (2022) 'Covid-19: Omicron sub variants driving new wave of infections in UK', *BMJ*, 377: o1506. https://doi.org/10.1136/bmj.o1506

WMA (1964) 'WMA declaration of Helsinki – ethical principles for medical research involving human subjects'. Available at: www.wma.net/policies-post/wma-declaration-of-helsinki-ethical-principles-for-medical-research-involving-human-subjects/ (accessed 16 August 2022).

Wood, A. J. et al. (2019) 'Good gig, bad gig: autonomy and algorithmic control in the global gig economy', *Work, Employment and Society*, 33(1): 56–75. https://doi.org/10.1177/0950017018785616

World Health Organization (2016) 'Guidance for managing ethical issues in infectious disease outbreaks'. Available at: apps.who.int/iris/handle/10665/250580 (accessed 16 August 2022).

Wymant, C. et al. (2021) 'The epidemiological impact of the NHS COVID-19 app', *Nature*, 594(7863): 408–412. https://doi.org/10.1038/s41586-021-03606-z

5

Data-driven decision-making beyond COVID-19: incorporating the voice of the child

Claire Bessant and Rachel Allsopp

Data-driven decision-making has been central to the UK government's response to the coronavirus (COVID-19) pandemic. In February 2021, the government memorably promoted a 'data not dates' approach to pandemic decision-making (Prime Minister's Office, 2021), describing its use of data as 'a cornerstone of the nation's fight against Coronavirus' (Department for Digital, Culture, Media and Sport (DCMS), 2021: 6). Indeed, during the pandemic the government utilised a range of data-driven approaches, from entirely automated, AI-powered processing to more 'mundane' uses of digital information and statistics to inform decisions (OMDDAC, 2021: 6).

In November 2020, Northumbria University and the Royal United Services Institute joined forces, forming the Arts and Humanities Research Council (AHRC)-funded Observatory for Monitoring Data-Driven Approaches to COVID-19 (OMDDAC) to monitor key developments in this area.[1] OMDDAC has since highlighted several important legal, ethical, regulatory and policy challenges resulting from the UK government's data-driven response, identifying key lessons to be learned to inform responses to related challenges in future (OMDDAC, 2021).

Early in 2021, OMDDAC identified that a critical perspective was missing from discussions of data-driven approaches to COVID-19: the voice of the child.[2] Children have been described as 'the hidden victims of COVID-19' (Barnardo's, 2021). Government decisions, including key decisions to introduce lockdowns and self-isolation requirements, have had a significant impact upon children, yet children's voices appear to have been excluded from discussions regarding the data-driven coronavirus response

(Children's Commissioner for England, 2020; Barnardo's, 2021). Although others have explored how the pandemic affected adults' views about governmental use of their data (Lewandowsky et al., 2021), the study discussed in this chapter is the first to recognise that children hold views on this important issue. Indeed, while it might not be considered surprising that children should have views about data-driven decision-making and should express those views when asked to do so, the need to explore children's views about governmental use of their data appears never to have been considered before the pandemic.

OMDDAC commissioned a child rights organisation, Investing in Children (IiC),[3] to seek children's views about how their data were being used during the pandemic. IiC used their innovative agenda day™ method, together with an online survey, to ask seventeen children their views about the UK government's data-driven approach to coronavirus. A crucial finding of this study was that many of these children considered the government had afforded their views insufficient consideration; a perspective reflected elsewhere (Barnardo's, 2021; Girlguiding, 2021; Lundy et al., 2021).

Increasingly, decisions impacting individuals are being determined based upon 'the data' (Lupton and Williamson, 2017; Barassi, 2020). Where decisions affect children, there may be a still greater reliance upon data, because children themselves are often viewed as incapable of contributing meaningfully to debates about matters affecting them (Barassi, 2019). During the pandemic, decisions made upon the basis of 'the data' resulted in lockdowns. Reliance upon data also led to a host of other data-driven decisions (to close schools, to determine exam results via algorithms) which impacted upon children's health, wellbeing and education in a way that adults may not have fully considered or perhaps could not have foreseen.

Before the coronavirus pandemic, some children had already expressed concern that their views and interests were not being considered by politicians, stating that they 'felt side-lined by adults making decisions without them' (Children's Commissioner for England, 2019: 1–2). The significant, negative impact of the government's pandemic decision-making upon children, the government's reliance upon data and a corresponding failure to consider the views and interests of affected children (resulting from a predisposition to ignore children's rights) appear to have magnified the existing issues, leaving many children feeling they had not been respected as citizens (#Covidunder19, 2020).

A key lesson to be learned from the pandemic is that policymakers could do more to respect children's interests, rights and views. To support this contention, this chapter first details the rights and interests of children impacted by the government's data-driven pandemic response. It considers why the increasing datafication of children requires children's views to be fed into data policy and explains why continued public sector data-driven decision-making post-pandemic is likely to result in the increasing marginalisation of children's voices in all policy areas. It subsequently presents the findings of OMDDAC's study, exploring children's perspectives through their own words. It highlights that the government's international obligations under the United Nations Convention on the Rights of the Child, including the obligation to afford children a right to be heard, do 'not cease in situations of crisis or in their aftermath' (United Nations Committee on the Rights of the Child (hereafter, UN Committee), 2009: para. 125). It suggests how the government could ensure children's views are incorporated into policy, both in times of emergency and more generally.

The government's data-driven pandemic response and its implications for children

Public and private sector bodies are increasingly using data, including individuals' personal data, to take data-driven decisions which affect our lives (Barassi, 2020; Robertson and Tisdall, 2020). The use of personal data in data-driven decision-making has been particularly evident during the coronavirus pandemic. The sharing of personal data from multiple sources (NHS Test and Trace datasets, the NHS list of patients for those who were shielding, general practitioner records, and local authority records regarding school attendance and free school meal eligibility) was crucial to supporting vulnerable individuals and delivering localised pandemic responses (London Councils, 2020; OMDDAC, 2021). Free school meals data was vital in ensuring free computers reached disadvantaged children (Department for Education, 2020). Novel approaches to data sharing were illustrated in public-private collaborations, resulting in prioritisation of supermarket delivery slots for vulnerable people (DCMS, 2021). In addition, statistical data (infection rate data and reproduction number (R number) data) were key to anticipating and understanding the spread of COVID-19, determining alert levels and deciding when to impose lockdowns (UK Health Security Agency, 2021a). Data on COVID-19 prevalence, COVID-19 vaccine deployment and health system capacity were key to determining the nature and severity of restrictions upon movement and social gatherings (Cabinet Office, 2021). Key technological data-driven innovations include the QCovid™ algorithm, which uses data to profile and identify people at high risk of hospitalisation, and the NHS COVID-19 app, a digital proximity app which identifies and notifies people who have been in close contact with someone who has contracted COVID-19 (Dawda et al., 2021).

While the government contends that data-driven decision-making played a vital role in addressing the pandemic (DCMS, 2020), the negative implications of the government's decisions for children must be acknowledged. Although children are at a reduced risk of becoming seriously ill from COVID-19, 'the secondary impacts of the pandemic', namely the government's data-driven decisions to impose restrictions and to close schools, have severely affected children (Children's Commissioner for England, 2020: 15).

In response to the pandemic, between late March 2020 and mid-July 2021, a series of national and local coronavirus regulations and directions were implemented, placing restrictions on individuals' movement and their ability to gather (Brown and Kirk-Wade, 2021). The United Kingdom entered its first national lockdown in late March 2020; everyone was ordered to stay at home, schools were closed to all but 'vulnerable children' and the children of 'key workers' (Cabinet Office and Department for Education, 2020). Most children, unable to attend school, were reliant upon schools providing remote or online learning. Many parents reported, however, that during this first lockdown their children's schools failed to provide any remote learning (OFQUAL, 2021). When further national lockdowns ensued in November 2020 and January 2021, again school attendance was limited to vulnerable children and critical workers' children (Department for Education, 2021).[4] Although there is some evidence that by January 2021 the quality of remote teaching had improved compared with during the first lockdown, many pupils were still unable to access online learning because they had no laptop (OFQUAL, 2021).

National lockdowns and social distancing requirements affected children's ability to socialise with friends and family (Streetgames, 2020), restricting their right to freedom of association (pursuant to Article 15 of the UN Convention on the Rights of the Child (UNCRC) and Article 11 of the European Convention on Human Rights (ECHR)). The Article 31 UNCRC right to leisure, play and recreation was hampered by lockdowns and the closure of schools and playgrounds (Children's Commissioner for England, 2020). Reduced physical activity, and loneliness caused by social isolation, had significant negative impacts upon children's ability to attain the highest standards of physical and mental health, protected by Article 24 of the UNCRC (Children's Commissioner for England, 2020: 15; Barnardo's, 2021; Young Minds, undated). Compounding matters, the NHS's capacity to treat children declined (Children's Commissioner for England, 2020; Barnardo's, 2021). Government-mandated school closures also had a severe impact upon children's ability to access an effective education (pursuant to Articles 28 and 29 of the UNCRC and Article 2, First Protocol of the ECHR), with pre-existing educational inequalities between children of richer and poorer households exacerbated (Barnardo's, 2021; Lundy et al., 2021).

While the principle of non-discrimination lies at the heart of the UNCRC (Article 2), the government's decisions have impacted most harshly upon those children already vulnerable to breaches of their rights (Children's Commissioner for England, 2020; Barnardo's, 2021; Lundy et al., 2021), particularly poorer children and children from black and minority ethnic (BAME) backgrounds.[5] The poor and disadvantaged were most likely to experience increased levels of violence and abuse, notwithstanding Article 19 UNCRC's right to protection from abuse and violence (Children's Commissioner for England, 2020; Lundy et al., 2021). Lockdowns had a catastrophic impact on family finances, pushing some families into poverty, with some struggling to pay bills and to feed their children

(Barnardo's, 2021), impacting upon children's Article 27 UNCRC right to an adequate standard of living. This has led some to describe the coronavirus pandemic as a 'syndemic' ('where the virus interacts with pre-existing vulnerabilities' that are 'driven by larger political, economic, social, and environmental processes') (Wernli et al. and Geneva Science Policy Interface, 2021: 4).

Children's privacy[6] was also affected by requirements for those testing positive for COVID-19 to provide contact information to NHS Test and Trace (UK Health Security Agency, 2020) and by schools obliging pupils to inform them when they tested positive (Cumbria County Council, undated). The use of algorithms to determine children's exam grades in August 2020 provides a final example of how data-driven decision-making affected children, again impacting most upon disadvantaged children (House of Commons Education Committee, 2020). With the majority of children prevented from attending school, and thus unable to sit examinations, the UK's qualification regulators[7] were directed to develop an alternative approach to awarding grades (Office for Statistics Regulation, 2021). In England, OFQUAL asked schools to provide the grade they thought a student would have received had their exams taken place. This information was combined with other data, including previous grades attained by students at each school and teacher-awarded grades for other 2020 exam candidates. When results were published, 40 per cent of grades had been moderated down by OFQUAL's algorithm (Children's Commissioner for England, 2020). Many children were unaware of the regulators' proposed alternative grading process, subsequently expressing concern about how their grades were calculated, the impact it had upon their ability to attend their desired university, and thus upon their futures (Busby, 2020; Priestley et al., 2020).

The UNCRC imposes significant obligations upon the UK, including requirements to treat the child's best interests as a primary consideration (Article 3). Every law and regulation that affects children should be underpinned by the 'best interests' criterion (UN Committee, 2013). During the pandemic, however, many decisions impacted negatively upon children, raising questions about the UK's compliance with Article 3 UNCRC (best interests) and Article 2 UNCRC (non-discrimination). Concerns have also been expressed about governmental failures to consult with children during the pandemic upon issues directly affecting them, and about the inability of decision-making processes 'to meaningfully respect children's rights to be active participants in decisions made about them' (Observatory of Children's Human Rights Scotland and Children and Young People's Commissioner Scotland, 2020: 5, 13). Article 12 UNCRC stipulates that 'States Parties shall assure to the child who is capable of forming his/her own views the right to express those views freely in matters affecting them, such views being given due weight in accordance with the age and maturity of the child'. Children themselves argue that to protect children's rights, children's voices must be heard (Office of the Special Representative of the Secretary-General on Violence Against Children, 2021), yet during the pandemic children have not felt heard; they have felt forgotten (Barnardo's, 2021; Girlguiding, 2021; Lundy et al., 2021). England's Children's Commissioner has suggested that during the pandemic children's best interests were not the government's primary consideration. Instead, children's needs were 'side-lined and ignored' and their rights 'downgraded' (Children's Commissioner for England, 2020: 27).

It is, of course, possible to argue that both the undue impact on children and lack of engagement with them are symptomatic of the same problem, that children's wellbeing and rights could not be prioritised during a pandemic where many basic human rights were suspended. Eminent child-rights scholars make clear, however, that such an argument is unsustainable. The UN Committee emphasises that children's views should be sought whenever their views are likely to improve the quality of the solutions (UN Committee, 2009: para. 27). It confirms that the Article 12 UNCRC right to be heard 'does not cease in situations of crisis or in their aftermath' (UN Committee, 2009: para. 125). Indeed, as Lundy et al. note, 'States' responses to the Covid-19 pandemic is one of the situations where there were (and are) clear and grave consequences for children's enjoyment of their human rights, and thus an obligation to engage with them quickly and directly' (Lundy et al., 2021: 262). Given that children's rights (e.g., to health, to protection from harm, to education, to play) were so significantly impacted, it is arguable that children were impacted by the pandemic more significantly than adults, and that there was, therefore, a crucial need to seek children's views.

A continued emphasis on data-driven decision-making and the 'datafication of children'

The UK government now proposes to build on its data-driven response to the coronavirus pandemic, suggesting a data-driven approach will be used to inform other 'governmental priorities, such as improving outcomes in education' (DCMS, 2021: 103). The government does not outline how such expanded data use may affect children, and there is no evidence that children's views have been sought either upon the government's Data Strategy (DCMS, 2020), or upon its proposals for data protection reform (DCMS, 2021).

Such a continued lack of focus on children is unsurprising. Policy debates tend often to be dominated by adults and by the view that young people need to be protected (Coleman et al., 2017; Barassi, 2019). The need to consider how data-driven decision-making impacts upon children is, however, more important now than ever. Children are 'increasingly datafied', through mobile phones, social media and education software, with data generated often being used to monitor, evaluate and make decisions about them (Lupton and Williamson, 2017: 781). Such 'dataveillance' reconfigures children into 'digital data assemblages'; once transformed 'into data' they are then used as 'numbers to influence or act on individuals' (Lupton and Williamson, 2017: 783). Consider, for instance, how during the pandemic individuals who tested positive for COVID-19, who were hospitalised, or who died became 'data' used to justify decisions to introduce lockdowns and to close schools.

Such 'dataveillance' raises important rights issues for children. Lupton and Williamson identify that increasingly data that 'speak for themselves' are being used 'in ways that override the rights of children to speak for themselves'; they suggest data-processing algorithms are 'erasing children's own embodied experiences and voices from decision-making processes' and that '[r]ather than engag[ing] children in their right to involvement in decisions about important matters that affect their lives, many analytics systems appear to distribute decision-making to automated, proprietary systems' (Lupton and Williamson, 2017: 790). They argue that in

> many approaches to the datafication and dataveillance of children, the embodied and subjective voices of children are displaced by

the supposed impartial objectivity provided by the technological mouthpieces of data. Data are positioned to provide a more detailed and manageable account of who children really are, free from the messiness of dialogic deliberation and freedom of expression.
(Lupton and Williamson, 2017: 790)

The study

Given the significant impact data-driven decision-making has had upon children, the indications such a data-driven approach will continue after the coronavirus pandemic, and the implications for children of such data-driven decision-making, OMDDAC decided to commission IiC to seek children's views on the government's data-driven response to the coronavirus pandemic.

Investing in Children

IiC is a children's human rights organisation which supports children to enter into dialogue with adult decision-makers.[8] IiC believes 'children are knowledgeable about the world in which they live and can be powerful participants in political dialogue and persuasive advocates on their own behalf' (IiC, undated-a).

IiC used its innovative, agenda day™ method to engage children in discussion.[9] An agenda day is an adult-free space. Child facilitators lead group conversations, encouraging other children to express views (Stalford et al., 2017; IiC, undated-b). Children themselves take primary responsibility for notetaking and report writing, although an IiC project worker assists, discussing issues for exploration prior to the agenda day, providing support where needed. Child facilitators and attendees all receive a nominal fee to thank them for their time.

Although agenda days traditionally take place in person, social distancing measures made a face-to-face event impossible. A virtual agenda day was therefore facilitated via Zoom, taking place on the evening of 7 July 2021, a time chosen to suit children. Conscious that many children were feeling 'Zoomed out', IiC also offered children the opportunity to contribute views via an online survey available from 23 June to 16 July 2021. The framework for the study was provided in a detailed brief, designed by OMDDAC.

Participants were recruited by IiC via email and Twitter. Recruitment was timed to ensure children's views could be incorporated into OMDDAC's final report (OMDDAC, 2021) and shared with policymakers. In accordance with Northumbria University ethics requirements and IiC procedures, consent was obtained from participants or their parents, depending upon age, using a consent form IiC co-produced with children.

In total, seventeen children participated. Five children aged 15–18, including two participant facilitators attended the agenda day. Twelve children completed the survey: two aged 11–13, five aged 14–16 and five aged 17–18. Children lived in areas ranked in deciles 3, 4, 5, 7 and 8 of the English Index of Multiple Deprivation (IMD), decile 1 encompassing the most deprived areas and decile 10 the least deprived (Ministry of Housing, Communities and Local Government, 2019).

The OMDDAC brief

OMDDAC's brief to IiC included open and closed questions, offering children the opportunity to respond to specific queries and provide more detailed commentary. The brief was designed to be accessible to children from primary school age upwards and relevant to policymakers. It contained several broad topics, which were explored at the agenda day and via the survey:

- what the children knew about how the government was responding to coronavirus; including what they knew about how information and technology were being used;
- from where they obtained their information;
- whether they wanted more information about the government's approach;
- whether they felt there had been enough discussion with them about data-driven decision-making;
- whether they would have liked their views to have been sought before decisions were made; and
- how they thought the government could obtain their views.

In addition, the brief covered three scenarios involving data-driven approaches used during the pandemic: wastewater testing; algorithmic determination of school grades; and monitoring of self-isolation obligations by police. The facilitators suggested the agenda day focus on two scenarios. Scenario 3 (police monitoring) was therefore not discussed at the agenda day, although it was included in the online survey.

The impact of algorithmic assessment of school grades is discussed above, as are the self-isolation requirements which prevented children from attending school and leisure activities. OMDDAC also decided to explore children's views on the less-discussed topic of wastewater analysis, having identified that this novel dataset was being used during the pandemic in unprecedented, innovative ways to detect geographical outbreaks of COVID-19 and inform local and national responses (Allsopp et al., 2021; OMDDAC, 2021; UK Health Security Agency, 2021b). Such testing is expected to continue post-pandemic, to monitor and respond to public health concerns but also, for example, to detect the presence of illegal substances (Ott, 2020; Van der Sloot, 2021). Academics are already raising concerns about potential 'scope creep', suggesting 'sewage monitoring might become one of the most common and invasive forms of surveillance' (Van der Sloot, 2021: 1). Including wastewater analysis in the brief afforded children a valuable opportunity to contribute their views to dialogue on this emerging issue.

Reflections on the study design

This study did not aim to achieve representativeness. The challenges of recruiting children as participants are widely recognised (Cree et al., 2002). Discussions with a large research consultancy suggest the challenges have been exacerbated during the pandemic. This study sought to investigate whether any children knew how data were being used in response to the pandemic, and to gain insights into children's views about such data use. Children themselves believe they can provide meaningful insights into issues which adults consider of limited importance (Office of the Special Representative of the Secretary-General on Violence Against Children, 2021). Academics suggest even small samples can afford valuable information about children's perspectives and experiences and can be useful in the development of practical recommendations (Millward and Senker, 2012).

The pandemic undoubtedly posed challenges. Social distancing measures meant some form of online engagement was the only realistic option. Using two different online data collection methods raised further issues. While individualised responses were provided by survey respondents, the agenda day report delivered a broader overview of discussions, as interpreted by the child facilitators. Agenda day participants only covered the first two scenarios, while survey respondents provided views on all three. Despite the recognised limitations of this study, the clear, often detailed, comments provided by the children nonetheless merit further consideration.

Findings

Several themes were identifiable from participants' comments. Specifically, the children wanted to be provided with reliable information about matters affecting them, including use of their data. They held clear views about how their data should be used, and they wanted to express those views and for the government to consider them.

Children want to be reliably informed

Most participants (five agenda day attendees, nine survey respondents) were aware of key measures introduced to address coronavirus (COVID-19), mentioning: lockdowns; social distancing; mandatory mask wearing; COVID-19 vaccinations; tiered travel restrictions; school closures; funded tutoring; monitoring of infection rate, hospitalisation and mortality data; NHS Test and Trace; and the NHS COVID-19 app. Gaps in knowledge were, nonetheless, evident. Answering the question 'What have the Government done to tackle COVID-19', one survey respondent said they did not know, two respondents failed to answer. Some agenda day attendees knew wastewater was being tested, others were 'absolutely clueless'. Seven survey respondents were unaware of wastewater testing. Awareness of the algorithms used to grade students again varied. All children attending the agenda day knew about the plans; seven survey respondents did not. Significantly, this included five children aged 14–18. This did not mean, however, that the children had no opinion about this proposal; indeed, all agenda day attendees and four survey respondents said they disliked the idea.

As to how children obtained information, the children referred to various avenues: schools, social media, parents, family, friends and televised and reported news.[10] Nonetheless, the children did not all believe they had received sufficient, trustworthy information from the government; five survey respondents thought children had been given insufficient information about government decisions relating to coronavirus, with one child commenting that policies 'aren't broadcasted well enough'. Although agenda day participants had seen official government announcements about coronavirus restrictions, this was through social media. They commented critically upon the government website: 'The Government has not used their website effectively as it was very difficult to read and understand. The young people were rather critical of the Government website as it was difficult to navigate.' This criticism is particularly notable given that agenda day attendees expressed concerns about the reliability of information gained from other sources, such as 'biased' news reporting and social media, which they described as 'a very untrustworthy source'.[11] Responses suggest even digitally literate children, who wish to keep themselves informed, may not always be able to effectively access government messaging, and that the government could do more to afford children access to information about policies affecting them.[12] Article 17 UNCRC (the right to access information and mass media) and Article 13 UNCRC (imposing an obligation on states 'to refrain from interfering in children's expression of their views, or in their access to information') are viewed as 'crucial prerequisites for the effective exercise' of the child's Article 12 UNCRC right to be heard (UN Committee, 2009: para. 80). Where children do not know how their data are used, or how decisions affecting them are made, they may be unable to effectively exercise their Article 12 UNCRC right. The importance of ensuring information is presented to children in child-friendly, understandable language is recognised nationally and internationally (UN Committee, 2009; Council of Europe, 2018; Information Commissioner's Office, 2020). In the context of data-driven decision-making, Article 12 of the UK General Data Protection Regulation (UKGDPR), further affords a right to receive information about the collection and processing of one's personal data. UKGDPR Article 12 and Recital 58 emphasise that information provided to children should be intelligible, easily accessible and in clear, plain language.

Children have views about the government's data-driven approach

Participants expressed clear, but mixed, views about the data-driven pandemic response. Ten did not support the education regulators' decision to use an algorithm to determine student grades, raising concerns about the inability of computers to determine a student's capabilities, as well as the exacerbation of a social class divide. One thought it a good plan, six were undecided. In relation to wastewater monitoring, again, views varied. The child facilitators in their agenda day report for example, described wastewater testing as 'innovative', explaining that agenda day attendees:

> believed that if it was going to protect people that it shouldn't matter if they felt that it was a little invasive as it is for the greater good. They said that it was a good way of identifying the COVID-19 hotpots. The young people didn't believe it to be an invasion of privacy because it could help prevent the spread of COVID-19 by recognising where most cases were and putting certain restrictions in place, such as a local lockdown.

Six survey respondents also considered wastewater testing an acceptable response. Two, however, were unsure. A further four opposed testing, with one stating, 'people need to be aware and consenting'. When asked whether information derived from such testing should be shared with others, again views varied. Agenda day attendees accepted the need to share data with health professionals and the local authority but were less happy for it to be shared with the police, elaborating that 'the police had no business in knowing this information' and querying 'what they would do in protecting the public with this information'. Several survey respondents thought it acceptable for the information to be widely shared, with two children suggesting it might even be shared publicly. Again, however, a preference was shown for sharing with health professionals and the local authority over the police (nine survey respondents supported information sharing with health professionals and the local council; five agreed to information sharing with the police). This aligns with findings from OMDDAC's nationally representative UK public perceptions survey, which also identified that adults were less prepared to share information with the police than with health professionals or local authorities (Sutton et al., 2021). Both this study and the adult public perceptions survey found also that participants were more willing to share anonymised information than non-anonymised information.

As mentioned above, agenda day attendees did not consider police monitoring. Survey respondents' views about the police being told when individuals are required to self-isolate were again divided. Five children considered disclosure acceptable; four were unsure; three objected. More children (eight) expressed concern, however, when asked how they would feel if *their family* were monitored to ensure they were self-isolating. Two children raised specific concerns about the police, one suggesting 'police are corrupt and have biases which could lead to unequal fines', the other worrying that any fines levied for non-compliance would 'disproportionately impact poorer families who often have no choice but to go to work'.

Overall comments suggest further research exploring children's views about public sector data sharing with the police would be valuable. Given the children's apparent lack of trust in the police, consideration should be given to exploring, with children, how trust in the police and other public bodies can be improved. The diversity and complexity of participants' views indicate a potential need for wider scale, representative research exploring children's views about public sector data-driven decision-making. Limited attention has been given to children's views about governmental use of their data (Milkaite et al., 2021; Stoilova et al., 2021). The only other study which considers children and data-driven decision-making focuses primarily upon children's data literacy, not children's views about governmental or public sector use of their data (Robertson and Tisdall, 2020).

Children want their views to be considered

The key message articulated by participants was that the government (not just academia) should consider their views. Seven survey respondents said there had been insufficient discussion with children.

Seven respondents also said young people should have been asked before decisions were taken about important matters such as school closures, COVID-19 testing at school and mask wearing at school. The agenda day report similarly illustrates the children's desire to feed into decision-making:

> Without any hesitation, definitely the young people would have wanted to be asked about the decisions being made, as it was their future so they should have a say. They said that if they were asked about wearing masks they would have agreed in a heartbeat as they would rather wear a mask than work on a laptop virtually at home.

Agenda day attendees clearly thought the government could have done more to engage with children and ensure their interests were considered, commenting that:

> young people are not considered enough, especially when the pandemic has affected them massively. People doing exams this year and last year, such as GCSEs weren't even considered when forming a plan and making big decisions about their futures. ... The young people seem frustrated as their futures have not been considered at all, they believe that COVID-19 is going to impact future employment and the government has simply ignored this.

Recommendations beyond COVID-19

As this chapter illustrates,

> [d]uring crises, every decision taken by governments not only affects the adults ... but ... has an impact on the community that surrounds children. ... It becomes important to seek children's views not only because of the direct implications that decisions during crises have, but also because there are numerous indirect impacts of such crises on children. (Lundy et al., 2021: 280)

It is widely recognised, however, that, as children in OMDDAC's study noted, during the coronavirus (COVID-19) pandemic children's views were absent from 'adult-centric' public discourse (Lundy et al., 2021), and those formulating policy solutions ignored children's interests in favour of adult concerns (Reid et al., 2022). Some academics recommend that policymakers should, in future, use Children's Rights

Impact Assessments to examine the potential impact on children of proposed laws, policies and decisions as they are developed, to avoid or mitigate negative impacts (Reid et al., 2022). Given the comments of the children who participated in OMDDAC's study, and given the government's UNCRC obligations, particularly under Article 12, it is suggested that the UK government should also incorporate children's views into policy- and decision-making, in times of emergency but also more generally. Such an approach accords with the UN's 2030 Agenda for Sustainable Development, which articulates member states' commitment to empower vulnerable people including children and makes explicit the role children may play as 'critical agents of change' (United Nations, undated: para. 51). Specifically, given its stated intention to continue its data-driven approach, the government should support children to become active agents in data policy. While it is often assumed that children lack the maturity and capacity to formulate opinions on such complex issues, OMDDAC's study challenges this view.

Children's participation and Article 12 UNCRC

Article 12 UNCRC is a particularly important right for children, because it affords children the status of rights holders entitled to participate in decision-making (Cuevas-Parra, 2021: 83). The UN Committee explains the term 'participation'

> is now widely used to describe ongoing processes, which include information sharing and dialogue between children and adults based on mutual respect, and in which children can learn how their views and those of adults are taken into account and shape the outcome of such processes. (UN Committee, 2009: para. 3)[13]

Effective, meaningful participation cannot, therefore, be understood as an individual one-off event (UN Committee, 2009: para. 133). Participation should involve two-way dialogue. It should be 'undertaken with the very specific purpose of enabling children to influence decision-making and bring about change' (Sinclair, 2004: 111).

Lundy's internationally respected model of participation, which reflects the UN Committee's understanding of how Article 12's obligations can be satisfied, is recommended as a basis for ensuring policy is informed by children's views (Lundy, 2007).[14] It comprises four components which form part of an iterative process of consultation, feedback and consultation:

1. **Space:** Children must be given the opportunity to express a view;
2. **Voice:** Children must be facilitated to express their views;
3. **Audience:** The view must be listened to; and
4. **Influence:** The view must be acted upon, as appropriate. (Lundy, 2007: 933)

Compliance with Article 2 UNCRC (non-discrimination) requires that any participation strategy acknowledges that children are not a homogeneous group (as illustrated by the diverse views expressed by study participants). Care must be taken to include perspectives from minority groups, including: home-schooled children, children excluded from or truanting from school, children in local authority care, children with disabilities, children for whom English is not a first language, children from travelling or socially excluded communities, and children from ethnic minority backgrounds (Borland et al., 2001). Materials must be child-friendly, multilingual, age- and capacity-appropriate and accessible to all children. This is particularly relevant given the negative comments expressed by participants concerning the government website.

Engagement methods

The children involved in OMDDAC's study suggested a range of methods government and policymakers might use to engage with children: through schools, youth organisations, social media and surveys, including surveys disseminated through schools. Further options include: one-to-one interviews; group discussions; interactive events; online discussions; events and conferences; consultation documents circulated for written comment; online consultation; visual approaches including maps and flow diagrams; video; theatre; formal structures such as youth forums and representative councils; youth juries; and face-to-face meetings between children and politicians (Borland et al., 2001; Coleman et al., 2017; Livingstone et al., 2019; Observatory of Children's Human Rights Scotland and Children and Young People's Commissioner Scotland, 2020; Barnardo's, 2021).

Many of these methods require careful thought for several reasons: the formal written consultation typically used by government departments[15] may be inaccessible to children, particularly those with disabilities or poor literacy; individual interviews are costly; and focus groups, group interviews, events and conferences, while popular with children, may inhibit marginalised and less vocal children from expressing their opinions. While the pandemic has illustrated the effectiveness and accessibility of large-scale online surveys designed with and for children, some investment may be needed to ensure children can interact safely with decision-makers via accessible, multilingual, age-appropriate digital platforms (Children's Commissioner for Wales, 2020; Children's Parliament, 2020; Girlguiding, 2021; Office of the Special Representative of the Secretary-General on Violence Against Children, 2021). Since not all children can access information technology (Joining Forces for All Children, 2021), some children may require support to complete surveys at school or college (Borland et al., 2001). A combination of methods may be required to ensure all children can express a view.

Crucially, many initiatives developed during the pandemic have illustrated the important role child- and youth-led organisations can play in supporting participation and in engaging 'hard-to-reach' children (Observatory of Children's Human Rights Scotland and Children and Young People's Commissioner Scotland, 2020; Office of the Special Representative of the Secretary-General on Violence Against Children, 2021). Children can provide invaluable advice upon the design of child-friendly resources (Stalford et al., 2017) and should be involved in the design and delivery of all communications to children (Observatory of Children's Human Rights Scotland and Children and Young People's Commissioner Scotland, 2020), particularly communications conveying 'often opaque' information about data processing (Milkaite et al., 2021: 6). Children, where trained, can also play an important role in identifying issues and collecting and analysing data from other children (Office of the Special Representative of the Secretary-General on Violence Against Children, 2021; Lundy et al., 2021). Ultimately, however, the government needs to invest in development of children's networks (Office of the Special Representative of the Secretary-General on Violence Against Children, 2021) and commit to resourcing and training individuals to engage with children: '[I]nvestment in the realization of the child's right to be heard in all matters of concern to her or him and for her or his views to be given due consideration, is a clear and immediate legal obligation of States parties under the Convention' (UN Committee, 2009: para. 135).

Listening to, hearing and acting upon children's views

Finally, and as Lundy's model recognises, it is not sufficient to simply ask children to provide their views. Effective participation requires the government to listen to and act on children's views. To ensure that children's rights and interests are protected, a shift in perception is needed from children as 'passive objects in need of protection' to 'active participants in decision making processes affecting them' (Observatory of Children's Human Rights Scotland and Children and Young People's Commissioner Scotland, 2020: 13). As the UN Committee recognises, this may 'necessitate dismantling the legal, political, economic, social and cultural barriers that currently impede children's opportunity to be heard and their access to participation in all matters affecting them. It requires a preparedness to challenge assumptions about children's capacities' (UN Committee, 2009: para. 135). If the lessons of the pandemic are to be learned, and acted on, political environments, structures and institutions must become 'more respectful of and responsive to children's civic society' (Joining Forces for All Children, 2021: 11).

Concluding comments

The coronavirus (COVID-19) pandemic, and the data-driven decisions taken in response, affected every aspect of children's lives. They are likely to have a long-lasting impact upon children (Irwin et al., 2022). Such obvious impacts mobilised researchers (including OMDDAC), the Children's Commissioners, NGOs and charities to seek children's views. Children's concerns that they have not been listened to have been expressed loudly across a plethora of projects and surveys,[16] including the study discussed in this chapter; a study which emphasises that many children are articulate, intelligent, want to, and when provided with appropriate information can, play a valuable role in responding to policies which impact upon children.

Of course, the pandemic brought unprecedented challenges for governments. One could argue that they did the best they could, that they could not be expected to take everyone's interests into account, that the UK government's approach, to make the protection of lives and livelihoods its 'overriding goal' (Cabinet Office, 2021) was the correct one. Such arguments are, however, ill-founded. As Lundy notes, the coronavirus pandemic was 'one of the situations where there were … clear and grave consequences for children's enjoyment of their human rights, and thus an obligation to engage with them quickly and directly' (Lundy et al., 2021: 262). UNCRC obligations continue to apply even 'in situations of crisis' (UN Committee, 2009: para. 125). The government's commitment to the UNCRC (Article 3) required it to treat children's best interests as a primary consideration, and to afford children a right to be heard.

During the pandemic, however, children faced a 'double-whammy' – a pre-existing preference for adults to take decisions without considering the child's perspective, a preference based upon misguided assumptions that children are incapable of contributing effectively to decision-making, and a data-driven approach to pandemic decision-making which encouraged the further marginalisation of children's views and rights. It has been suggested that data are often assumed to speak for themselves (Lupton and Williamson, 2017: 790). As the eminent statistician, David Spiegelhalter, highlighted during the pandemic, however, '[d]ata does not speak for itself – it needs people to speak honestly and carefully on its behalf' (Spiegelhalter and Masters, 2022). Where decisions affect children, children need to be afforded the opportunity to express their views. Indeed, children make clear that where (data-driven) decisions are taken without additional reference being made to those affected, such decisions may not only have a negative impact on them, but may also result in them feeling that they are not afforded due respect as citizens (#Covidunder19, 2020).

Pre-pandemic, many of the concerns about the dataveillance of children have focused upon commercial organisations and technologies. The UK government's data-driven pandemic response, and its assertions that it will continue and develop this data-driven approach post-pandemic in areas affecting children, now require us to turn renewed attention to state dataveillance, the impact of governmental data-driven decision-making upon children, and how children's views are fed into decision-making. The coronavirus emergency and the government's response has made apparent the complex relationship between public sector data-driven decision-making and the child's UNCRC rights to be heard, to receive information and to have their best interests treated as a primary consideration. In this, the first study to have asked children about governmental use of data to make decisions affecting them, children's views are clear. They want to be listened to.

It is impossible to know whether outcomes/policy would have been different had the UK government and other governments listened to children. If governments had listened to children, they might still have come to the same conclusions. It is easy in hindsight to recognise where decisions have had significant negative impacts upon children. In the midst of the pandemic, it was perhaps less easy, for example, to identify the long-term impact of school closures. The fact that decisions might have been the same does not mean that it was not still important to listen to children. They have a right to be listened to and their views taken into account.

In any future pandemic, governments must be mindful of the views expressed by children during this pandemic and, respecting their obligations under the UNCRC, pay careful attention to their rights and interests. As important, the UK government should act now to ensure children's UNCRC rights are fully recognised and that, in accordance with the recommendations made in this chapter, its approach to decision-making is informed not only by data but also by children's views and interests.

Notes

1 See www.omddac.org.uk/ (accessed 21 September 2022).
2 In this chapter, the term 'children' encompasses all children and young people under the age of eighteen, reflecting the terminology in Article 1 United Nations Convention on the Rights of the Child (UNCRC).
3 See https://investinginchildren.net/ (accessed 24 August 2022).
4 Reclassification from key to critical workers (parents whose work was critical either to the coronavirus or EU transition response) meant

more children attended school in the second and third lockdowns, albeit most continued to access education remotely. See: https://educationhub.blog.gov.uk/2021/01/08/am-i-a-critical-worker-or-are-they-vulnerable-or-without-internet-access-or-broadband/

5 Children's access to public green space for play was limited, especially in poorer urban areas. Eight per cent of children in England had no access to a private garden, rising to 22 per cent for children from BAME backgrounds (Children's Commissioner for England, 2020: 24).

6 Protected by Article 16 UNCRC and European Convention on Human Rights Article 8.

7 In England, the Office of Qualifications and Examinations Regulation (OFQUAL); in Scotland, Scottish Qualifications Authority (SQA); in Wales, Qualifications Wales; in Northern Ireland, Council for the Curriculum, Examinations & Assessment (CCEA).

8 https://investinginchildren.net/ (accessed 24 August 2022).

9 An approach used in the UK, and internationally (by Irish Child and Family Agency, Tusla (www.tusla.ie/uploads/content/Investing_in_Children_Agenda_Days_2021.pdf) and by Norwegian children's rights organisation Med Ungdom in Fokus (https://ungdom.com/).

10 These sources are similar to those other children report using (Children's Commissioner for Wales, 2020; Children's Parliament, 2020).

11 Other children have expressed similar concerns about social media (Lundy et al., 2021).

12 Also suggested by other children (Children's Parliament, 2020).

13 For detailed discussion of what effective participation entails, see Bessant (2022).

14 Lundy's model has been used nationally and internationally to give children a voice (Department of Children and Youth Affairs, 2015; Leicester City Council, undated; World Health Organization, 2018).

15 For example, the consultation document, 'Data: a new direction' (DCMS, 2021).

16 See, for example: Children's Commissioner, 2020; Barnardo's, 2021; Girlguiding, 2021; United Nations Special Representative of the Secretary General on Violence Against Children, undated; #CovidUnder19, 2020.

References

#Covidunder19 (2020) 'Children's rights during coronavirus: children's views and experiences'. Available at: www.tdh.org/en/digital-library/documents/covidunder19-life-under-coronavirus-results-of-the-survey (accessed 4 November 2022).

Allsopp, R. et al. (2021) 'Snapshot Report 1: data-driven public policy', OMDDAC. Available at: www.omddac.org.uk/wp-content/uploads/2021/05/OMDDAC-Snapshot-Report-1-Public-Policy.pdf (accessed 24 August 2022).

Barassi, V. (2019) 'Datafied citizens in the age of coerced digital participation', *Sociological Research Online*, 24(3): 414–429. https://doi.org/10.1177/1360780419857734

Barassi, V. (2020) *Child Data Citizen: How Tech Companies Are Profiling Us from before Birth*, Cambridge, MA: MIT Press.

Barnardo's (2021) 'Supporting the hidden victims of COVID-19: lessons learned from the first wave'. Available at: www.barnardos.org.uk/sites/default/files/2021-02/supporting-hidden-victims-of-COVID-19.pdf (accessed 24 August 2022).

Bessant, C. (2022) 'Children, public sector data-driven decision-making and Article 12 UNCRC', *European Journal of Law and Technology*, 13(2). Available at: https://ejlt.org/index.php/ejlt/article/view/872

Borland, M. et al. (2001) 'Improving consultation with children and young people in relevant aspects of policy-making and legislation in Scotland', *SP Paper* 365. Available at: https://archive.scottish.parliament.uk/business/committees/historic/education/reports-01/edconsultrep01.htm#P178_2693 (accessed 4 November 2022).

Brown, J. and Kirk-Wade, E. (2021) 'Coronavirus: a history of "lockdown laws" in England', HC Briefing Paper 9068. Available at: https://researchbriefings.files.parliament.uk/documents/CBP-9068/CBP-9068.pdf (accessed 4 November 2022).

Busby, M. (2020) 'A-level students speak: I always dreamed of going to Cambridge', *Guardian*, 15 August. Available at: www.theguardian.com/education/2020/aug/15/a-level-students-protest-at-classist-government-algorithm (accessed 21 September 2022).

Cabinet Office (2021) 'COVID-19 response – Spring 2021'. Available at: www.gov.uk/government/publications/covid-19-response-spring-2021/covid-19-response-spring-2021 (accessed 4 November 2022).

Cabinet Office and Department for Education (2020) 'Guidance: critical workers and vulnerable children who can access schools or educational settings'. Available at: https://webarchive.nationalarchives.gov.uk/ukgwa/20210104165629/https://www.gov.uk/government/publications/coronavirus-covid-19-maintaining-educational-provision/guidance-for-schools-colleges-and-local-authorities-on-maintaining-educational-provision (accessed 4 November 2022).

Children's Commissioner for England (2019) 'Children's insights: what they do and think'. Available at: www.childrenscommissioner.gov.uk/wp-content/uploads/2019/10/CC_Childrens-Insights_issue1_30.10.pdf (accessed 4 November 2022).

Children's Commissioner for England (2020) 'Childhood in the time of COVID'. Available at: www.childrenscommissioner.gov.uk/wp-content/uploads/2020/09/cco-childhood-in-the-time-of-COVID.pdf (accessed 21 September 2022).

Children's Commissioner for Wales (2020) 'Coronavirus and me'. Available at: www.childcomwales.org.uk/wp-content/uploads/2020/06/FINAL_formattedCVRep_EN.pdf (accessed 24 August 2022).

Children's Parliament (2020) 'Finding out how children get news and information about the pandemic – and checking in on learning and health', *Corona Times Journal*, 5. Available at: www.childrensparliament.org.uk/childrens-journal-5/ (accessed 24 August 2022).

Coleman, S. et al. (2017) 'The Internet on our own terms: how children and young people deliberated about their digital rights'. Available at: https://5rightsfoundation.com/static/Internet-On-Our-Own-Terms.pdf (accessed 24 August 2022).

Council of Europe (2018) *Guidelines to Respect, Protect and Fulfil the Rights of the Child in the Digital Environment. Recommendation CM/Rec (2018) 7 of the Committee of Ministers*. Available at: https://rm.coe.int/guidelines-to-respect-protect-and-fulfil-the-rights-of-the-child-in-th/16808d881a (accessed 24 August 2022).

Cree, V. E., Kay, H. and Tisdall, K. (2002) 'Research with children: sharing the dilemmas', *Child and Family Social Work*, 7(1): 47–56. https://doi.org/10.1046/j.1365-2206.2002.00223.x

Cuevas-Parra, P. (2021) 'Thirty years after the UNCRC: children and young people's participation continues to struggle in a COVID-19 world', *Journal of Social Welfare and Family Law*, 43(1): 81–98. https://doi.org/10.1080/09649069.2021.1876309

Cumbria County Council (undated) 'Coronavirus (COVID-19) – information for schools and early year settings'. Available at: www.cumbria.gov.uk/coronavirus/education.asp (accessed 21 September 2022).

Dawda, S. et al. (2021) 'Snapshot Report 2: tech-driven approaches to public health', OMDDAC. Available at: www.omddac.org.uk/wp-content/uploads/2021/05/OMDDAC-Snapshot-Report-2-Tech-Driven-Approaches-to-Public-Health.pdf (accessed 21 September 2022).

DCMS (Department for Digital, Culture, Media & Sport) (2020) 'UK national data strategy'. Available at: www.gov.uk/government/publications/uk-national-data-strategy/national-data-strategy (accessed 24 August 2022).

DCMS (Department for Digital, Culture, Media & Sport) (2021) 'Data: a new direction'. Available at: www.gov.uk/government/consultations/data-a-new-direction (accessed 24 August 2022).

Department for Education (2020) 'Devices and connectivity provided to disadvantaged children and young people'. Available at: https://get-help-with-tech.education.gov.uk/devices/device-allocations (accessed 21 September 2022).

Department for Education (2021) 'Get the facts about vulnerable and critical worker children', *The Education Hub Blog*, 8 January. Available at: https://educationhub.blog.gov.uk/2021/01/08/am-i-a-critical-worker-or-are-they-vulnerable-or-without-internet-access-or-broadband/ (accessed 4 November 2022).

Department of Children and Youth Affairs (2015) 'National strategy on children and young people's participation in decision-making, 2015–2020', Dublin: Government Publications. Available at: https://assets.gov.ie/24462/48a6f98a921446ad85829585389e57de.pdf (accessed 22 July 2022).

Girlguiding (2021) 'Girls' attitudes survey 2021'. Available at: www.girlguiding.org.uk/globalassets/docs-and-resources/research-and-campaigns/girls-attitudes-survey-2021-report.pdf (accessed 24 August 2022).

House of Commons Education Committee (2020) 'Getting the grades they've earned. COVID-19: the cancellation of exams and "calculated" grades', First Report of Session 2019–21 (HC 617). Available at: https://committees.parliament.uk/publications/1834/documents/17976/default/ (accessed 4 November 2022).

Information Commissioner's Office (2020) 'Age appropriate design: a code of practice for online services'. Available at: https://ico.org.uk/media/for-organisations/guide-to-data-protection/ico-codes-of-practice/age-appropriate-design-a-code-of-practice-for-online-services-2-1.pdf (accessed 24 August 2022).

Investing in Children (undated-a) 'Our history'. Available at: https://investinginchildren.net/?page_id=247323 (accessed 24 August 2022).

Investing in Children (undated-b) 'What we do'. Available at: https://investinginchildren.net/?page_id=42 (accessed 22 September 2022).

Irwin, M. et al. (2022) 'The COVID-19 pandemic and its potential enduring impact on children', *Current Opinion in Pediatrics*, 34(1): 107–115. https://doi.org/10.1097/MOP.0000000000001097

Joining Forces for All Children (2021) 'Children's right to be heard: We're talking, are you listening?' Available at: https://joining-forces.org/wp-content/uploads/2021/01/policy_brief-We_re_Talking-Are_You_Listening-EN.pdf (accessed 21 September 2022).

Leicester City Council (undated) 'Social care and education participation approach: ensuring children and young people realise their rights'. Available at: https://consultations.leicester.gov.uk/communications/yp-participation/results/youngpeopleparticipationstrategy.pdf (accessed 22 July 2022).

Lewandowsky, S. et al. (2021) 'Public acceptance of privacy-encroaching policies to address the COVID-19 pandemic in the United Kingdom', *PLoS ONE*, 16(1). https://doi.org/10.1371/journal.pone.0245740

Livingstone, S., Stoilova, M. and Nandagiri, R. (2019) 'Talking to children about data and privacy online: research methodology', London: London School of Economics and Political Science. Available at: www.lse.ac.uk/media-and-communications/assets/documents/research/projects/childrens-privacy-online/Talking-to-children-about-data-and-privacy-online-methodology-final.pdf (accessed 24 August 2022).

London Councils (2020) 'A London Council member briefing: London's health response to the pandemic'. Available at: www.londoncouncils.gov.uk/sites/default/files/London-Health-Response-to-COVID.pdf (accessed 21 September 2022).

Lundy, L. (2007) '"Voice" is not enough: conceptualising Article 12 of the United Nations Convention on the Rights of the Child', *British Educational Research Journal*, 33(6): 927–942.

Lundy, L. et al. (2021) 'Life under coronavirus: children's views on the experiences of their human rights', *International Journal of Children's Rights*, 29(2): 261–285. https://doi.org/10.1163/15718182-29020015

Lupton, D. and Williamson, B. (2017) 'The datafied child: the dataveillance of children and implications for their rights', *New Media & Society*, 19(5): 780–794. https://doi.org/10.1177/1461444816686328

Milkaite, I. et al. (2021) 'Children's reflections on privacy and the protection of their personal data: a child-centric approach to data protection information formats', *Children and Youth Services Reviews*, 129: 106170. https://doi.org/10.1016/j.childyouth.2021.106170

Millward, L. and Senker, S. (2012) 'Self-determination in rehabilitation: a qualitative case study of three young offenders on community orders', *British Journal of Forensic Practice*, 14(3): 204–216. https://doi.org/10.1108/14636641211254923

Ministry of Housing, Communities and Local Government (2019) 'English indices of deprivation 2019'. Available at: www.gov.uk/government/statistics/english-indices-of-deprivation-2019 (accessed 24 August 2022).

Observatory of Children's Human Rights Scotland and Children and Young People's Commissioner Scotland (2020) 'Independent children's rights impact assessment on the response to COVID-19 in Scotland'. Available at: https://cypcs.org.uk/wpcypcs/wp-content/uploads/2020/07/independent-cria.pdf (accessed 4 November 2022).

Office for Statistics Regulation (2021) 'Ensuring statistical models command public confidence: learning lessons from the approach to developing models for awarding grades in the UK in 2020'. Available at: https://osr.statisticsauthority.gov.uk/wp-content/uploads/2021/03/Ensuring_statistical_models_command_public_confidence.pdf (accessed 4 November 2022).

Office of the Special Representative of the Secretary-General on Violence Against Children (2021) 'Children as agents of positive change'. Available at: https://violenceagainstchildren.un.org/sites/violenceagainstchildren.un.org/files/documents/publications/children_as_agents_of_positive_change.pdf (accessed 4 November 2022).

OFQUAL (2021) 'Learning during the pandemic: review of research from England'. Available at: www.gov.uk/government/publications/learning-during-the-pandemic/learning-during-the-pandemic-review-of-research-from-england#the-impact-the-pandemic-has-had-on-learning (accessed 4 November 2022).

OMDDAC (2021) 'Final report: Data-driven responses to COVID-19: lessons learned', OMDDAC Research Compendium. Available at: www.omddac.org.uk/news/final-report-omddac-lessons-learned/ (accessed 24 August 2022).

Ott, A. (2020) 'Monitoring wastewater for COVID-19', UK Parliament, 15 December. Available at: https://post.parliament.uk/monitoring-wastewater-for-COVID-19/ (accessed 24 August 2022).

Priestley, M. et al. (2020) 'Rapid review of national qualifications experience 2020', Faculty of Social Sciences, University of Stirling. Available at: www.gov.scot/binaries/content/documents/govscot/publications/independent-report/2020/10/rapid-review-national-qualifications-experience-20202/documents/rapid-review-national-qualifications-experience-2020/rapid-review-national-qualifications-experience-2020/govscot%3Adocument/rapid-review-national-qualifications-experience-2020.pdf (accessed 4 November 2022).

Prime Minister's Office (2021) 'PM statement to the House of Commons on roadmap for easing lockdown restrictions in England: 22 February 2021'. Available at: www.gov.uk/government/speeches/pm-statement-to-the-house-of-commons-on-roadmap-for-easing-lockdown-restrictions-in-england-22-february-2021 (accessed 24 August 2022).

Reid, K., Tisdall, K. and Morrison, F. (2022) 'Children's rights impact assessments in times of crisis: learning from COVID-19', *International Journal of Children's Rights*. https://doi.org/10.1080/13642987.2022.2061955

Robertson, J. and Tisdall, K. (2020) 'The importance of consulting children and young people about data literacy', *Journal of Media Literacy Education*, 12(3): 58–74. https://doi.org/10.23860/JMLE-2020-12-3-6

Sinclair, R. (2004) 'Participation in practice: making it meaningful, effective and sustainable', *Children and Society*, 18: 106–118. https://doi.org/10.1002/chi.817

Spiegelhalter, D. and Masters, A. (2022) 'Can you capture the complex reality of the pandemic with numbers? Well, we tried', *Guardian*, 2 January. Available at: www.theguardian.com/commentisfree/2022/jan/02/2021-year-when-interpreting-covid-statistics-crucial-to-reach-truth (accessed 4 November 2022).

Stalford, H. et al. (2017) 'Achieving child friendly justice through child friendly methods: let's start with the right to information', *Social Inclusion*, 5(3): 207–218. https://doi.org/10.17645/si.v5i3.1043

Stoilova, M. et al. (2021) 'Children's understanding of personal data and privacy online: a systematic evidence mapping', *Information, Communication & Society*, 24(4): 557–575. https://doi.org/10.1080/1369118X.2019.1657164

Streetgames (2020) 'The experience of the coronavirus lockdown in low-income areas of England and Wales'. Available at: https://static1.squarespace.com/static/5f020c49b484e47001f2bb5b/t/5f725af9a49c1a4ec084df77/1601329934881/Coronavirus_report.pdf (accessed 21 September 2022).

Sutton, S. et al. (2021) 'Snapshot Report 4: survey of public perceptions of data sharing for COVID-19 related purposes', OMDDAC. Available at: www.omddac.org.uk/wp-content/uploads/2021/08/WP3-Snapshot. pdf (accessed 24 August 2022).

UK Health Security Agency (2020, updated 2021) 'NHS Test and Trace: what to do if you are contacted'. Available at: www.gov.uk/guidance/ nhs-test-and-trace-how-it-works (accessed 21 September 2022).

UK Health Security Agency (2021a) 'UK COVID-19 alert level methodology: an overview'. Available at: www.gov.uk/government/publications/ uk-COVID-19-alert-level-methodology-an-overview/uk-COVID-19-alert-level-methodology-an-overview (accessed 21 September 2022).

UK Health Security Agency (2021b) 'Wastewater testing coverage data for the Environmental Monitoring for Health Protection (EMHP) programme'. Available at: www.gov.uk/government/publications/ wastewater-testing-coverage-data-for-19-may-2021-emhp-programme/ wastewater-testing-coverage-data-for-the-environmental-monitoring-for-health-protection-emhp-programme (accessed 24 August 2022).

UN Committee (United Nations Committee on the Rights of the Child) (2009) *General Comment No. 12 (2009) The Right of the Child to be Heard*, 20 July 2009, CRC/C/GC/12. Geneva: United Nations. Available at: https://digitallibrary.un.org/record/671444?ln=en (accessed 4 November 2022).

UN Committee (United Nations Committee on the Rights of the Child) (2013) 'General comment No. 14 on the right of the child to have his or her best interests taken as a primary consideration', 29 May, CRC/C/GC/14. Geneva: United Nations. Available at: www2.ohchr.org/ English/bodies/crc/docs/GC/CRC_C_GC_14_ENG.pdf (accessed 4 November 2022).

United Nations (undated) 'Transforming our world: The 2030 Agenda for Sustainable Development', A/RES/70/1. Available at: https://sustainable development.un.org/content/documents/21252030%20Agenda%20 for%20Sustainable%20Development%20web.pdf (accessed 4 November 2022).

United Nations Special Representative of the Secretary General on Violence Against Children (undated) '#CovidUnder19: fulfilling children's right to be heard and participate in the response to the pandemic'. Available at: https://violenceagainstchildren.un.org/content/covidunder19 (accessed 4 November 2022).

Van der Sloot, B. (2021) 'Truth from the sewage: are we flushing privacy down the drain?', *European Journal of Law and Technology*, 12(3). Available at: https://ejlt.org/index.php/ejlt/article/view/766/1043

Wernli, D. et al. and Geneva Science Policy Interface (2021) 'Governance in the age of complexity: building resilience to COVID-19 and future pandemics'. Available at: www.leru.org/files/GSPI-PolicyBrief_resilience. pdf (accessed 4 November 2022).

World Health Organization (2018) 'Engaging young people for health and sustainable development: strategic opportunities for the World Health

Organization and partners'. Available at: https://apps.who.int/iris/bitstream/handle/10665/274368/9789241514576-eng.pdf?sequence=1&isAllowed=y (accessed 22 July 2022).

Young Minds (undated) 'The impact of COVID-19 on young people with mental health needs'. Available at: www.youngminds.org.uk/about-us/reports-and-impact/coronavirus-impact-on-young-people-with-mental-health-needs (accessed 21 September 2022).

6

Where are publics in pandemic public policy?

Jamie Webb and Kiran Kaur Manku

In this chapter we argue that when the UK government engaged publics during the coronavirus (COVID-19) pandemic, it did so in ways that reduced them to imagined publics or passive objects to be measured, rather than elevating them as active citizens whose values should be incorporated into decision-making.[1] To support this claim, we provide a brief survey of pandemic public engagement, contrasting the diverse range of activities conducted by non-central government agencies with the limited way the UK government engaged publics during the pandemic, remaining on the lower rungs of Sherry Arnstein's (1969) ladder of citizen participation (Figure 6.1).

We highlight how the narratives and policies deployed by the government actively removed values from policymaking and communication with publics. This reflected a hollowing out of values in policy, supposedly justified by the oft-repeated scientific mantra, 'follow the science' (GOV.UK, 2020: 8), an impossible guiding principle given the irreducible trade-offs governments face during a pandemic, but one which demonstrated a disinclination to engage with the plurality of values that publics would bring to policy questions.

This status quo posed a challenge for those who wished to engage publics more substantively in pandemic decision-making. In our experience, centring the perspectives of publics can uncover new questions, positions and values that may be neglected in their absence, particularly because of the epistemic benefits that engaging diverse non-expert publics can bring (Bohman, 2006; Landemore, 2013). This is a very different activity from providing direct guidance on the questions and policy challenges that decision-makers may already have formulated in the absence of engaging publics (Weible et al., 2012).

We explore this challenge through our own experiences of engaging publics and policymakers during the pandemic as researchers on the UK Pandemic Ethics Accelerator, an interdisciplinary and cross-institution ethics research group,[2] specifically through our work on the Accelerator's public dialogue and policy workshop. Our solution is to narrow this gap between policymakers and publics by institutionalising structures that allow publics more substantial deliberative engagement in policymaking. We follow the OECD (2020) in defining this institutionalisation as the incorporation of deliberative activities into governance structures in a way that establishes a legal or regulatory framework to ensure continuity regardless of political change. A variety of institutionalised public engagement activities conducted outside of the UK government is considered, before challenges to effective institutionalisation are acknowledged. Despite these challenges, we recommend the institutionalisation of participatory forms of governance that centre ethical deliberation of public values in policy decisions.

An overview of pandemic public engagement

The breadth of engagement work conducted by UK organisations outside of central government during the coronavirus pandemic demonstrates the variety of methodologies, purposes and partnerships that can be employed for publics to participate in policymaking. The heterogeneity of these activities confounds any attempt at providing necessary and sufficient conditions for what makes something 'public engagement' (Webb, 2021b) but their overlapping features can be shown through case studies of work carried out during the pandemic.

Surveys, focus groups and workshops have all been used to gain a better understanding of public perspectives on key issues during the pandemic. For example, a 1,003-person survey inquired about views on coronavirus certification (Serco Institute, 2021), while another survey of over 2,000 UK adults investigated attitudes towards inequalities and coronavirus (Duffy et al., 2021). An online focus group was used to explore participant perceptions and experiences of social distancing and social isolation during the pandemic (Williams et al., 2020), while a dialogic workshop investigated attitudes towards vaccination among minoritised groups (Traverse, 2021).

Publics have also been involved in creating tools to help others manage through the pandemic: the CoRay project, led by Emerging Minds, worked with young people to develop and share their own resources for dealing with the disruption and challenges the pandemic brought (Emerging Minds, 2022). Partnerships have been devised between research institutes and publics, for example when Health Data Research UK (HDR UK) created an eighteen-person public panel to explore perspectives on making regional, linked health data available to support vaccine safety research (Slape, 2022). Elsewhere, the Scottish government crowdfunded ideas for the COVID-19 response from its citizens, allowing registered users to submit ideas, rate the ideas of other users, and provide (moderated) comments (Participedia, 2021c).

Even more radically, deliberative democracy has engaged representative groups of non-expert members of publics in learning from expert testimony, discussing, deliberating and making policy recommendations on pandemic issues, using deliberative bodies such as Citizens' Juries and larger Citizens' Assemblies. Cases in the UK include Citizens' Juries assembled to deliberate on the provision of scarce ICU resources (Kuylen et al., 2021), on the use of health data to combat the pandemic (Oswald and Laverty, 2021), and on building public trust in a contact tracing app (Ada Lovelace Institute, 2020). Deliberative approaches have also been used in devolved and local areas. A Citizens' Panel in Scotland was made part of the oversight of the Scottish government's coronavirus response (Participedia, 2021d). A Citizens' Assembly in Camden considered the impact of coronavirus on local residents (Participedia, 2021b), while one in Bristol set priorities for the city's pandemic recovery (Participedia, 2021a).

Inadequacies in UK government pandemic public engagement

This diverse array of public engagement activities conducted during the pandemic stands in stark contrast to the role of publics in the

UK government's decision-making at the beginning of the coronavirus pandemic. Major decisions were taken which rested on catastrophically false beliefs about the purported behaviour of a homogenised and imagined public. The choice to delay lockdown until 23 March 2020 was taken partly based on concerns of behavioural fatigue: the belief that the British public would never accept stringent lockdown measures for any significant length of time. This intuitive folk judgement – connecting exceptionalist narratives about freedom-loving Britons and the Orientalist assumption that what was possible with a supposedly pliable Chinese public would not be accepted here – was not based on any respected concept in behavioural science.[3] Rather it was an imagined public, created by politicians and scientific advisers, that shaped the space of conceivable policy decisions during the initial spread of coronavirus (Ballo et al., 2022: 11–12). In 2020, the most important political decision since the Second World War was guided by the same phenomenon that pragmatist philosopher, John Dewey, identified in 1927: 'our political "common-sense" philosophy imputes a public only to support and substantiate the behaviour of officials' (Dewey, 2016 [1927]: 150).

This could be excused as an unfortunate consequence of decision-making under conditions of extreme uncertainty, at the start of a pandemic which has often been described as unprecedented and unforeseeable.[4] However, since that point, the UK government's use of public engagement to inform policymaking was limited. Public engagement was used as a tool of measurement, as with surveys and opinion polls. Here, knowledge has been extracted from publics – for example, their attitudes towards social distancing requirements, their engagement with contact tracing, their willingness to get vaccinated, their support for vaccination certification, and so on – to inform policy decisions taken by government (ONS, 2023). It was also used to inform and influence publics in certain ways – for example, through public information campaigns informing people about social distancing rules or encouraging them to get vaccinated (PHE, 2021).

Referring to Sherry Arnstein's ladder of citizen participation (Arnstein, 1969: 217), government engagement operated at the level of what Arnstein identifies as 'tokenism' (see Figure 6.1). Informing publics, while a necessary first step to more substantive

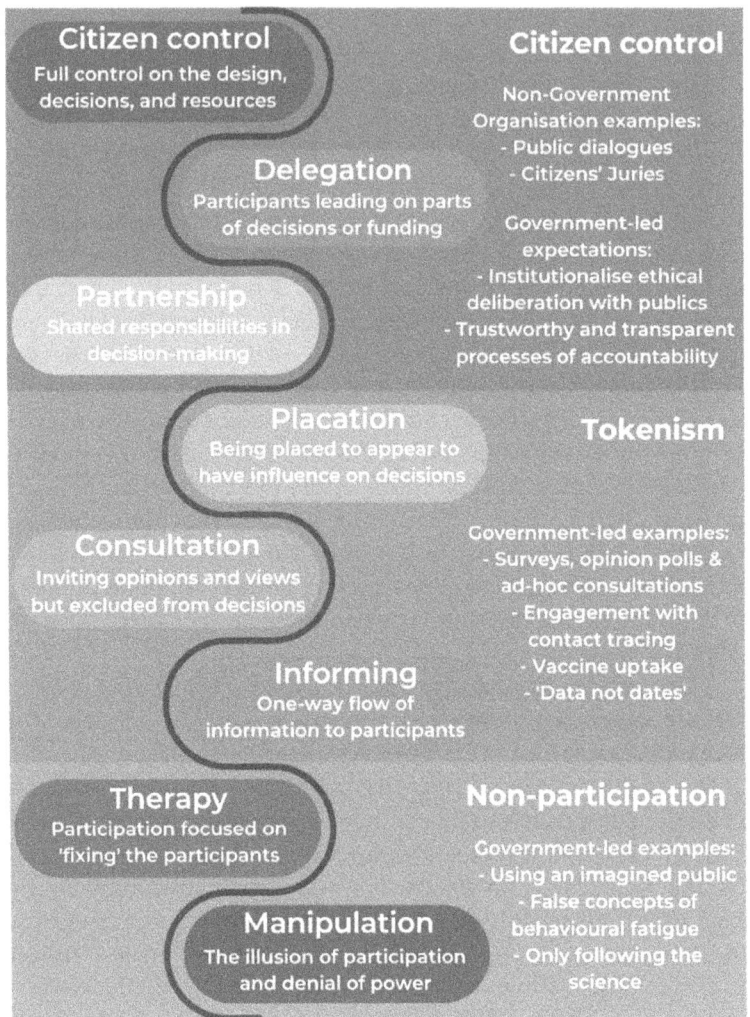

Figure 6.1 Arnstein's Ladder of Citizen Participation

participation, is often used as a one-way flow of information with limited opportunity for dialogue.[5] Through these engagements, publics are made passive and disconnected from any direct creative influence on the decisions that affect them or the wellbeing of their fellow citizens.

More substantive government-led engagement was rare. When it was sought – for example, the call for evidence regarding attitudes to COVID-19 vaccine mandates for care home workers – no explanation was provided in advance regarding how responses would be taken into account in the policy decision (GOV.UK, 2021). When in-depth interviews and focus groups were conducted with publics during the pandemic by the government and its opposition, the focus was often on overcoming barriers, that is, how to make an already agreed policy more palatable for citizens, or on perceptions and compliance with an agreed policy, for example social distancing guidance (Mavron, 2021). Citizens who engaged in these discussions were not given the power to *inform* policymaking, merely to offer a reaction. This accords with Arnstein's critique of 'tokenistic' consultation practices, which often operate as nothing more than window dressing, a façade of engagement with no real substantive impact (Arnstein, 1969: 217).

Further up the ladder comes partnership – where individuals are able to negotiate and engage in trade-offs with traditional power structures – and delegation and citizen control – where citizens occupy direct decision-making authority – all of which confer increasing degrees of citizen power (Arnstein, 1969: 217). The examples of public engagement conducted during the pandemic given at the start of this chapter demonstrate the wide variety of methodological approaches that can be leveraged to meet aspirations higher up this ladder. But this work was largely conducted by private organisations, academics, public and third sector bodies, or local and devolved authorities. Central government-led engagement never progressed above the lower rungs of the ladder.

The impossibility of value-free policymaking

This tokenistic engagement of publics was in keeping with the government's self-mythologised model of pandemic decision-making. The claim that government decision-making was 'guided by the science' was a constant refrain at Downing Street press briefings (GOV.UK, 2020), as was 'data not dates' in planning the lifting of coronavirus (COVID-19) restrictions (BBC News, 2021). These narratives legitimised the government's approach to engagement. In focusing on measurement and communication, they created a role for publics as a collection of atomised data points, made passive subjects of scientific instruction, to be assessed like lab measurements in a research study, not engaged in collective processes of decision-making. Non-expert publics lack scientific expertise, and, if our decision-making process is simply following an imagined scientific consensus, climbing higher up the ladder of citizen participation to more proactively engage citizens is not only unnecessary but an irresponsible waste of time and money.

Of course, these narratives were fictions, promoting a model of scientific deference that obscured the essentially value-laden nature of political decision-making: for example, the relative weighting of economic activity, personal freedom, public health and diverging pandemic risks to different demographic groups (Ballo et al., 2022: 6). Nevertheless, as well as creating a scientised model of their imagined public, this narrative encouraged a hollowing out of how value-laden decisions were made and communicated. Inescapably moral decisions that rested with government were either offloaded to others, hidden from sight, or reimagined as encompassing purely 'scientific' concerns. In late March 2020, for example, when COVID-19 threatened to overwhelm hospitals and necessitate triage decisions over ventilators and ICU beds, UK health officials rejected a draft guideline that proposed a scoring system incorporating age, frailty and comorbidities to guide allocation decisions (Kirkpatrick and Mueller, 2020). No official NHS guidance was produced, leaving decisions to local health authorities and individual doctors (Wilkinson et al., 2020). The membership of the Scientific Advisory Group for Emergencies (SAGE) and the minutes from its early meetings were kept secret until the end of May 2020. As a result (and, presumably, by design) the process of how scientific advice informed policy deliberations was made opaque to citizens in the crucial early stages of the pandemic (Freedman, 2020; Landler and Castle, 2020).[6] Furthermore, in advising on whether to recommend the vaccination of 12–15 year olds, the Joint Council of Vaccination and Immunisation (JCVI) explicitly limited itself to consideration of the direct benefits and risks of vaccination on the child being vaccinated (JCVI, 2021). Consideration of the broader societal impacts of vaccination were not delegated to any other official body, nor was an explanation provided for how they would be considered in government decision-making. Arguably, a general culture of opacity as to how values informed government pandemic decision-making facilitated the obscuring of some of the values informing specific behaviours: for example, greed and cronyism in the procurement of government contracts (Siddique, 2022), and the prioritisation of internal Conservative Party unity in the decision to lift COVID-19 restrictions (Riley-Smith and Knapton, 2022).

While government may still contend that it was accountable to citizens, this notion of accountability was devoid of any reference to ethical values. This was most obviously seen with Partygate,[7] as even government figures who accepted this behaviour was wrong claimed that the continuing focus on Partygate was a distraction from getting things done, which is what they said people 'really cared about' (Rogers, 2022). Further, a key contention was that, in any case, it was undemocratic for the Prime Minister to leave office over the scandal because of the majority the Conservative Party had won at the last election (Wingate, 2022). But Partygate was about the *moral conduct* of individuals in government, and people *did* care about what Partygate revealed about the ethics of people operating at the highest levels of public office (Ferguson, 2022). Restricting the ability of citizens to advocate for ethical standards in public life to a vote in the General Election every four years – when this vote must also be used to express policy preferences and pass judgement on the competence of their local candidates for MP – is, we argue, a massive hollowing out of ethics and public participation in governance.

The Hopkins Van Mil public dialogue

This reality – of limited government public engagement, ethically opaque policymaking, yet a strong independent evidence base of meaningful coronavirus (COVID-19) pandemic engagement activities – influenced our own public engagement work during the pandemic. The authors of this chapter were researchers on the UK Pandemic Ethics Accelerator (hereafter 'the Accelerator'), an interdisciplinary and cross-institution research group which worked to bring UK ethics research expertise to bear on the multiple, ongoing ethical challenges that arise during pandemics. The Accelerator aimed to provide rapid evidence, guidance and critical analysis to decision-makers across science, medicine, government and public health (Ethics Accelerator, 2022).

Both authors were primarily attached to the Accelerator's 'public values, transparency and governance' workstream. As well as producing pieces of theoretical work – including ethical analysis of pandemic public engagement activities (Webb, 2021b), a tracker of public engagement work conducted during the pandemic (Webb, 2022) and an analysis of the ethical arguments provided by Conservative MPs against COVID-19 certification (Webb, 2021a) – this work stream aimed to directly engage publics and policymakers in the ethical challenges that arose during the pandemic.

Building on our analysis of pandemic public engagement work, we entered the planning of our own engagement having made some explicit methodological choices. Rather than measuring or predicting the beliefs or preferences of publics to gauge support for a proposed policy choice, we wanted to give space to participants to explore the relationship between their ethical values and the coronavirus response. This took us higher up Arnstein's ladder of participation (Figure 6.1), and required a methodological approach aimed at facilitating dialogue and deliberation among participants. This explicitly ruled out opinion polls or surveys as methods. The Accelerator therefore commissioned the public engagement firm Hopkins Van Mil (HVM) to lead a public dialogue. HVM specialises in encouraging engagement through social research techniques to design, facilitate and report on approaches including dialogue, focus groups and community mapping (HVM, 2023).

Although this was only a small-scale public dialogue with twenty-four people from across the UK invited to take part, a specification and screener were used to ensure that the group reflected a diverse segment of the UK population, including guaranteeing a range of different locations: urban, suburban, rural and coastal (HVM, 2021: 6). This was important because a major epistemic benefit of representativeness is that publics bring a diversity of experiences and expertise to discussions (Bohman, 2006; Landemore, 2013). Representativeness can lead to the inclusion of a broader range of ethical values than the usual risk-benefit calculations espoused by many experts, considering a range of social and practical considerations that impact on those affected by policymaking.[8]

Where are publics in pandemic public policy? 133

We further reflected that many of the dialogic and deliberative events conducted in the UK during the pandemic, such as those detailed in the first part of this chapter, had a narrow, directed focus on a single issue or region. While the topics of dialogue in these events had clear ethical significance, public values were not always the explicit focus.[9] In contrast, we wanted to give participants a wide degree of freedom to *shape* the topics of discussion and what they viewed as the key ethical issues emerging during the pandemic. A primary motivation for doing this research was the desire to use the results to engage policymakers with the values of importance to participants, in a way that prior government-led engagement work had not done.

HVM convened three two-hour workshops during July and August 2021, with sessions focusing on participants' experiences with coronavirus, their priorities for the COVID-19 recovery, and how they believed the UK government should prepare for future pandemics. An online homeworking space was also in use before and during the dialogues, so that participants could watch informational videos, engage in online discussion and deliberation, and shape aspects of future workshop sessions.

A thorough summary of the processes and results of this engagement can be found in the HVM report 'Pandemic ethics: a public dialogue' (HVM, 2021). However, we wish here to briefly highlight some of the distinctive ethical perspectives participants brought to the engagement. Participants spoke candidly about their frustrations with the government's lack of recognition of the value-ladenness of decision-making – 'Not once have I heard anybody mention the ethical implications of going into lockdown' (HVM, 2021: 34) – and a desire for meaningful public engagement to meet this challenge: 'Let's get a policy built from that, so all of us can be involved' (HVM, 2021: 41).

Some participants were concerned that vaccines were not the all-protective shield they were sometimes presented as being (HVM, 2021: 16), and recommended extra steps be taken to protect the clinically vulnerable, including the destigmatisation of mask wearing (HVM, 2021: 21), increased capacity for home working (HVM, 2021: 24), and increased support for community healthcare (HVM, 2021: 27).[10] Many participants were sceptical of the return to normal promoted by the government (HVM, 2021: 20), and viewed the pandemic recovery as an opportunity to embrace new ways of living, with increased support for mental health (HVM, 2021: 22), research into long COVID (HVM, 2021: 23), and experiments in Universal Basic Income (HVM, 2021: 28–29). Finally, they examined issues through novel ethical lenses, considering safety (HVM, 2021: 33) and kindness (HVM, 2021: 26) as key ethical values, and over the course of the dialogue shifted from an initial focus on individual choice to a more collective response to adversity (HVM, 2021: 40).

The researchers at HVM highlighted several key priorities identified by participants as particularly important for the coronavirus recovery and future pandemic responses. They included the following:

- Re-balance inequalities that coronavirus exposed and exacerbated: address disparities in healthcare, particularly those experienced by people with Black, Asian and Minority Ethnic heritage, and combat poverty which worsened alongside intolerable inequalities.[11]
- Build trust and transparency into government policies and actions: for example, through greater collaboration across the home nations to provide consistent and clear messaging and communications for citizens across the UK.
- Develop public involvement in policymaking: to create a society which is resilient in the face of future pandemics, participants want ordinary citizens to be involved in shaping future policies (HVM, 2021: 2–3).

The Westminster policy workshop

Following the publication of the dialogue report in September 2021, the Accelerator hosted a workshop in the Houses of Parliament to engage policymakers, advocate for greater public engagement in ethical policymaking, and showcase the results of the dialogue. The logistical challenges of securing a venue in parliament, our desire to invite a wide variety of stakeholders, and the need to organise a high-quality programme and set of speakers, meant the workshop took place in May 2022. It engaged forty parliamentarians, policymakers, patient representatives and academics.

The ordering of events so that the public dialogue led into the policy workshop was designed intentionally to centre the outcome of the public dialogue in the aims of the workshop. Rather than centring the interests of policymakers, and having the questions they wanted to consider determine the content of the dialogue, we wanted the priorities and values of participants to be prioritised and decide the content of the policy workshop.

This was achieved in several ways. First, one-page summaries of the results of the HVM dialogue were distributed to attendees in information packs at the event. Second, the topics chosen to structure the event, and therefore influencing the choice of invited speakers and the content of the discussions, were taken directly from the priorities identified by dialogue participants. The first half of the event focused on addressing inequalities, and the second on trust and transparency. Both parts of the event involved one speaker directly describing the views of participants on those issues. Third, several speakers, including one of the authors of this chapter, made direct calls for more radical forms of participatory engagement to be institutionalised in pandemic policymaking (something for which dialogue participants had also expressed a desire).

Despite the clear methodological justification for doing things 'this way round', it is important to note the difficulties of this approach. One of the challenges of influencing policymakers is the need to meet them where they are: both physically – which is why we wanted to hold the event in the heart of government – and in the delivery of information, by providing specific content designed to fit their evolving agenda. A common objection to academics' attempts to influence political decision-makers is that the former leave the latter with new questions, new problems and new complications, but few concrete solutions or suggestions as to how decision-makers should respond to the challenges they face. As Weible et al. point out in their widely cited paper on public policy, goal achievement in policy influencing often requires attention to issues within an *existing* government programme or policy (Weible et al., 2012: 6). Academics who wish to have a demonstrable impact on public policy are, therefore, often advised first to find out what problems policymakers face and want guidance on, and then to provide direct answers to those questions.

This is a particular challenge given the kind of ethical expertise we were attempting to provide to policymakers. Knowledge can come in two forms, either propositional or performative (Archard, 2011). Propositional knowledge is knowledge that something is the case, whereas performative knowledge is an understanding of how to enact or engage in a process. Propositional moral knowledge was not the form of ethical expertise that we wished the policy workshop to consider. Rather, we wanted to highlight the range of ethical factors that we argue must be weighed in pandemic policy decisions, and advocate for a long-term procedural shift where more power was given to the deliberations of publics as a key part of the performance of this weighing process. We wanted to give publics the opportunity to pose their own questions and develop their own solutions to the problems they have identified. It was observing a lack of opportunities for non-expert publics to have this kind of input in pandemic policymaking that motivated the HVM dialogue and our methodological choices. But this kind of engagement is less likely to receive uptake in policymaking, because, instead of producing results already tailored to the immediate policy problems of decision-makers in positions of power, it may suggest different priorities altogether.

It is, therefore, possible that our workshop might have had more chance of directly impacting policy if we had done things 'the other way round', with the topics of the workshop being set by policymakers, and with the speakers providing their responses to these predetermined topics. But this would have taken control away from the participants whom we wished to empower. This tension is potentially irresolvable within the current policy landscape. It would only be resolved by a significant redistribution of power from the executive branch of central government (revealed by the pandemic to be the main source of decision-making authority) to publics assembled to discuss, deliberate and, crucially, to *inform decisions*. A central aim of our workshops was to advocate for that approach, to try to create the conditions from within which our dialogue and its deliberations would seem a natural and essential component of policymaking.

A further challenge with engaging policymakers in a workshop specifically focused on ethics is that they are afforded relatively few opportunities for structured discussion and deliberation on ethical values. This can be seen in the ethical opacity of the UK's COVID-19 policies, and the way ethical values were missing in 'follow the science' narratives, as described in the opening part of this chapter. It was also seen through discussions at the policy workshop. One attendee[12] described being asked to provide ethical input into the government's decision of whether to introduce COVID-19 vaccine certification, but upon submitting their report, being asked to remove the references to 'solidarity' within the document.[13] The reluctance on the part of government to consider ethical values was reflected in the relative novelty, more than two years into the pandemic, of having an event in Westminster explicitly focus on pandemic ethics.

Key points emerging from our workshop were a call for explicit engagement with the ethical tensions of pandemic decision-making through trustworthy processes, including engaging publics on these matters of ethical value. The Accelerator offered support for this work through sharing tools to help approach ethically complex decisions in fast changing situations and build capacity to ensure ethics is at the centre of organisational decision-making. A summary of the workshop was produced, distributed directly to all participants, and published online (Manku, 2022).

The workshop was well received, with positive engagement during and after the event. It provided an opportunity to build relationships with policymakers, many of whom wanted to engage with the Accelerator further. Given that the objectives arising from the workshop – particularly the need to effect procedural changes to embed ethics and public involvement into decision-making – can only properly be met in the long term, prolonged engagement with policymakers will be essential in securing them. However, the standard fixed-term funding model of projects like the Accelerator means that longitudinal engagement from within a single research initiative is a particular challenge. The maximum length for UKRI-funded coronavirus-specific projects was eighteen months (UKRI, 2020). The Accelerator officially concluded its research activities on 31 July 2022. Any further engagement that researchers on the project can facilitate with policymakers to meet the goals arising from the workshop can only be done as individuals, without access to the project infrastructure for resources and support.

Our experience was that the point at which we had begun to build significant relationships, crucial for developing ethics expertise, was also the point the project had to end. This funding model thus poses challenges to gaining the necessary recognition from policymakers for progress to be made. As Weible et al. (2012: 1) argue, successful policy engagement requires three factors: deep knowledge; building networks; and participation for extended periods of time. We were able to achieve the first two parts of this formula within the timespan of the Accelerator, but not the final one.

A final challenge was striking the balance between our work *outside* of governance processes, providing critique and modelling best practices, and that which made attempts, like the policy workshop, to directly influence policymakers and have an impact *within* the current political landscape. How best do we bring public ethics to policy: through modelling a constructive process from the outside or by trying to influence decisions from the inside? This is, in itself, a moral choice. The best chance of influencing policy entails moulding the advice to the needs of current decision-makers. It is hard to do that ethically when the behaviour of so many in the executive and ministerial positions of government has been shown to be *unethical*.

During the pandemic, there were multiple breaches of the Nolan Principles that are supposed to guide behaviour in public life (Oliver, 2021), and a revision of the ministerial code which failed to strengthen the enforcement of standards in government (Durrant, 2022). Prime Minister Rishi Sunak only appointed Sir Laurie Magnus as his government's ethics adviser in December 2022, over six months after the previous officeholder, Lord Christopher Geidt, resigned in June 2022, with two other prime ministers in that time having left the position vacant (BBC News, 2022). Prime Minister Sunak ignored the recommendations of the Committee on Standards in Public Life to give the adviser the authority to begin investigations into ministerial conduct without the authority of the prime minister (Brown, 2022). Furthermore, the only independent ethical body institutionalised within government, the Moral and Ethical Advisory Group (MEAG), which was set up in March 2020 at the start of the pandemic to provide the government with expert advice on ethical issues in health and social care, officially closed in October 2022, following its last meeting in December 2021 (GOV.UK, 2022). The short-lived nature of MEAG's tenure is not a sign of a government committed to proactively engaging with the ethical aspects of its own policymaking.

The attendees at our policy workshop all demonstrated a great commitment to integrating ethics into public life. But they were self-selecting. Those most in need of heeding the messages of the workshop were probably not in attendance. Unfortunately, at this moment in public life, they are the ones most likely to be wielding the greatest power.

Recommendations

How might these issues be addressed? There is no simple way to bridge the gap between modelling participatory governance and having internal influence on policymaking. One approach is through sustained modelling of best practice by non-government organisations. This approach enables reputations of competence to be built with sympathetic politicians or policymakers with power – which may be at a local or devolved level – as a foundation for integrating those best practices into decision-making structures. During the workshop, Simon Burall, one of our panellists and a director at the public engagement company Involve, spoke about his own recent experiences with Camden Council using participatory methods to design and implement a Data Charter, engaging local residents in deciding how their data should be used to deliver public services (Involve, 2022).[14] This level of sustained engagement may not be possible for projects supported by short-term research grants, such as the Accelerator. But this would not be so great a problem if practices of participatory democracy were integrated into long-term decision-making structures, so that their presence would not remain dependent on sympathetic politicians and policymakers, who may be replaced by less sympathetic successors through the democratic process. Properly institutionalising participatory democracy would allow short-term research projects to utilise existing structures to engage publics on particular questions rather than justify, create and promote an infrastructure from scratch each time.

Institutionalising participatory governance could also address two of the challenges recognised during our work: the gap between the challenges policymakers face and the perspectives of publics. By recentring ethical discussion and deliberation about public values within policy decisions, the gap between the policymakers and publics would be bridged, and value judgements of publics would be integrated into decision-making from the outset. Experts who then engaged with policymakers on the pressing questions facing them would do so on the basis of their already having been informed by public deliberation. Our experience of the HVM dialogue indicates that those discussions would involve a plurality of sophisticated ethical perspectives grounded in the lived realities of ordinary citizens, ensuring that policy decisions would not be so detached from ethical reasoning as they have been during the pandemic.[15]

But what could this institutionalisation of public dialogue and deliberation look like in practice? Although it feels very far removed from how UK government decision-making operated during the pandemic, there are moves from governments across the world to use approaches from far higher up Arnstein's ladder of participation to integrate the perspectives of their citizens. Taiwan is an excellent example of the potential for mass participation deliberative approaches. It used online platforms to great effect during the pandemic to mobilise citizens in the fight against COVID-19 (Nabben, 2021). Taiwanese citizens were engaged in information gathering, discussion and deliberation which directly informed decision-making: an egalitarian vision of technology-facilitated democracy. A Citizens' Council has been made a formal part of government structures in Paris (Sortition Foundation, 2021) as has a Citizens' Assembly on climate in Brussels (G1000, 2022). The EU's Conference on the Future of Europe involved four panels of 200 European citizens from the twenty-seven member states, chosen through random selection (EU, 2022). This led to the European Commission committing to institutionalise European Citizens' Panels (ECPs) as a regular part of consultations prior to major legislative proposals (Greubel, 2022).

There are opportunities to be similarly bold in the UK, where local examples such as the development of Camden Council's Data Charter could be scaled up to a national level. In 2022, Labour unveiled plans for House of Lords reform, committing to a consultation on whether it should be replaced with an elected second chamber (Mason and Brooks, 2022). These plans were scaled back in 2023 (Helm and Savage, 2023). But even if an elected chamber were introduced, it is possible that it would be just as unresponsive to the perspectives, values and arguments of ordinary citizens as the democratically elected members of the UK government were during the coronavirus crisis. To fully elevate citizens up Arnstein's ladder, a representative body of citizens assembled through sortition to deliberate on ethically laden policy decisions could become an institutionalised part of government decision-making.

These proposals are radical, and we accept they must be embarked upon carefully and with an awareness of the challenges they face. The Conservative government did not show a desire to engage publics higher up Arnstein's ladder of participation during the pandemic. As such support is an important ingredient in securing institutionalised public engagement (Cornwall, 2004), the case for it must be made as strong as possible. Though this reputation has been severely tarnished in recent years, the government is expected to provide expertise and competence in decision-making. To create the best case for reform, efforts to institutionalise public deliberation should follow established best practice in order to ensure transparency, trustworthiness, and accountability to citizens (Chwalisz, 2021). Participatory work must always have its motivations explicitly conveyed, its methodologies justified, and its results properly contextualised.

Institutionalisation is still in the experimental stage (OECD, 2020). Even where it has seemed most successful, follow through is not guaranteed. Iceland's 2010–13 constitutional process, which engaged a representative Constitutional Assembly to review its constitution, led to a revised text which won the support of 67 per cent of voters in a non-binding referendum. But efforts to enshrine it in law were abandoned following the succession of a new government (Landemore, 2020). Early participatory budgeting initiatives in Brazil, which particularly focused on the preferences of poor and minoritised citizens, and led to a greater acknowledgement of their needs in municipal spending priorities, have been held up as a great success of public deliberation. However, over time, the level of political endorsement for participatory budgeting waned, leading to its ultimate discontinuation in its birthplace of Porto Alegre in 2017 (Abers et al., 2018). The challenges of building a more radically participatory democracy are very real. The case for its long-lasting institutionalisation in the UK must be made now, then again as it is established, and then again, and again, long into the future.

Conclusion

This chapter has shown that publics have only been permitted a passive, disengaged role in public policymaking during the COVID-19 pandemic: policymaking that has too often failed to grapple with ethical values. Nevertheless, examples of more participatory engagement demonstrate that involving publics and ethics in policymaking is possible. To realise this potential, we conducted our own public dialogue and brought its results to policymakers. Although the Accelerator's main work is now completed, we as individual researchers will continue to advocate for the role of ethics in public life, and for a more radically participative role for publics in ethical deliberations to inform public policy.

Notes

1 We use 'publics' rather than 'the public' throughout this chapter because there is no single monolithic public that can be surveyed, engaged or deliberated with. Instead, publics are constructed through different methods of engagement, and their characteristics and capabilities determined by this construction (Felt and Fochler, 2010). Using the term 'public' would obscure the active process of constructing publics that has occurred throughout the pandemic. The use of 'public values' at points throughout this chapter should not be taken as a suggestion that there are fixed values all citizens share, but that more participatory and representative forms of engagement can be used to involve publics in dialogue and deliberation on policy decisions so that their ethical perspectives, informed by this process of engagement, can be accounted for in decision-making.
2 The Accelerator's website and research outputs can be found at: https://ukpandemicethics.org/
3 Some later survey findings suggested this belief in a freedom-loving British public was not just false, but comically so. A survey into public attitudes towards the closure of various types of businesses during the pandemic found that 26 per cent of respondents were supportive of the closure of all nightclubs, *even when there was no threat of coronavirus at all* (Skinner, 2021).
4 Putting aside the fact that a zoonotic pandemic had been widely anticipated and the UK had been previously assessed as having the second highest level of pandemic preparedness in the world (Cameron et al., 2019).

5 Though Arnstein does not explicitly consider measurement as a form of participation, this has been pursued by the UK government as a method of engagement likewise characterised by one-way information flow – with information moving from measured publics to the government, but in a process controlled by government, with no channel for more participatory engagement to follow from it.
6 This early opacity was a major factor in the decision to form Independent SAGE so that scientific advice was transparently available to citizens (Landler and Castle, 2020).
7 A political scandal involving parties held by government staff during the pandemic while public health restrictions meant social distancing rules were in place which prohibited most gatherings: see BBC News (2023) for a timeline of events.
8 For example, a Canadian public deliberation on colorectal cancer screening recommendations found particular participant concerns around the level of information regarding screening options that would be provided to patients, and vulnerability within the doctor–patient relationship if a patient resisted screening. These factors had not been considered by an expert panel which focused its analysis more narrowly on clinical benefits and cost-effectiveness (Solomon and Abelson, 2012).
9 A clear exception to this general rule was the deliberative event on prioritisation of ICU resource allocation, which revealed considered prioritisation preferences balancing the ethical values of efficiency, vulnerability and equality. Our approach differed in that we wanted participants to shape the topics for discussion and deliberation rather than be directed to consider one particular topic, in this case the allocation of scarce resources in an ICU (Kuylen et al., 2021).
10 This collection of suggestions was reminiscent of the 'Swiss cheese model' in pandemic management, where multiple layers of risk management strategies are used to build more resilient health systems, in contrast to the government's approach of removing protective measures as part of their 'living with covid' strategy (Williams and Michie, 2022).
11 For more discussion on inequalities, coronavirus and the coronavirus recovery, see Marmot et al. (2020). For a project on the experiences of Black and Asian healthcare staff during the pandemic, see Ramamurthy et al. (2022).
12 This comment has been anonymised in accordance with the event being run along Chatham House Rules, where reporting of participants' contributions is permitted provided these contributions are not attributed to any particular individual at the event.
13 Solidarity can be defined as the enacted commitment to carry the 'costs' (financial, social, emotional and other contributions) of

assisting others with whom a person(s) recognises similarity in a relevant respect (Prainsack and Buyx, 2017: 77).
14 This contribution to the workshop is attributed to Simon Burall with their permission.
15 Relatedly, the OECD list seven purported benefits of representative deliberative processes: they can lead to better policy outcome, give decision-makers greater legitimacy, enhance public trust, signal civic respect and empower citizens, make governance more inclusive, strengthen integrity and prevent corruption, and help counteract polarisation and disinformation (OECD, 2020: ch. 6).

References

Abers, R. et al. (2018) 'Porto Alegre: Participatory Budgeting and the Challenge of Sustaining Transformative Change'. World Resources Institute. Available at: www.wri.org/research/porto-alegre-participatory-budgeting-and-challenge-sustaining-transformative-change (accessed 19 July 2023).

Ada Lovelace Institute (2020) 'Confidence in a crisis? Building public trust in a contact tracing app'. Available at: www.adalovelaceinstitute.org/report/confidence-in-crisis-building-public-trust-contact-tracing-app/ (accessed 19 July 2023).

Archard, D. (2011) 'Why moral philosophers are not and should not be moral experts', *Bioethics*, 25(3): 119–127. https://doi.org/10.1111/j.1467-8519.2009.01748.x

Arnstein, S. (1969) 'A ladder of citizen participation', *Journal of the American Institute of Planners*, 35(4): 216–224. https://doi.org/10.1080/01944366908977225

Ballo, R. et al. (2022) 'Socially-distanced science: how British publics were imagined, modelled and marginalised in political and expert responses to the COVID-19 pandemic', *SocArXiv*. https://doi.org/10.31235/osf.io/jc82q

BBC News (2021) 'Covid: Boris Johnson to focus on "data, not dates" for lockdown easing'. Available at: www.bbc.com/news/uk-56095552 (accessed 19 July 2023).

BBC News (2022) 'No 10 publishes Lord Geidt resignation letter to PM'. Available at: www.bbc.com/news/uk-politics-61822998 (accessed 19 July 2023).

BBC News (2023) 'Partygate: a timeline of the lockdown parties'. Available at: www.bbc.com/news/uk-politics-59952395 (accessed 19 July 2023).

Bohman, J. (2006) 'Deliberative democracy and the epistemic benefits of diversity', *Episteme*, 3(3): 175–191. https://doi.org/10.3366/epi.2006.3.3.175

Brown, F. (2022) 'Rishi Sunak appoints head of Historic England as ethics adviser', *Sky News*. Available at: https://news.sky.com/story/rishi-sunak-appoints-head-of-historic-england-as-ethics-adviser-12773172 (accessed 19 July 2023).

Cameron, E., Nuzzo, J. and Bell, J. (2019) '2019 Global Health Security Index'. Johns Hopkins University, The Economist Intelligence Unit (EIU) and the Nuclear Health Initiative (NTI). Available at: www.ghsindex.org/wp-content/uploads/2019/10/2019-Global-Health-Security-Index.pdf (accessed 19 July 2023).

Chwalisz, C. (2021) 'Eight ways to institutionalise deliberative democracy'. OECD. Available at: www.oecd.org/gov/open-government/eight-ways-to-institutionalise-deliberative-democracy-overview.pdf (accessed 19 July 2023).

Cornwall, A. (2004) 'Introduction: new democratic spaces? The politics and dynamics of institutionalised participation', *IDS Bulletin*, 35: 1–10. https://doi.org/10.1111/j.1759-5436.2004.tb00115.x

Dewey, J. (2016 [1927]) *The Public and Its Problems: An Essay in Political Inquiry* (ed. M. L. Rogers), University Park, PA: Penn State University Press. Available at: www.jstor.org/stable/10.5325/j.ctt7v1gh

Duffy, B. et al. (2021) 'Unequal Britain: attitudes to inequalities after Covid-19', King's College London. https://doi.org/10.18742/PUB01-043

Durrant, T. (2022) 'The new ministerial code fails again to improve standards', *The Institute for Government*. Available at: www.instituteforgovernment.org.uk/blog/new-ministerial-code (accessed 19 July 2023).

Emerging Minds (2022) 'CoRAY Project'. Available at: https://emergingminds.org.uk/co-ray-project/ (accessed 19 July 2023).

Ethics Accelerator (2022) 'UK Pandemic Ethics Accelerator: about'. UK Pandemic Ethics Accelerator. Available at: https://ukpandemicethics.org/about/ (accessed 19 July 2023).

EU (2022) 'European Citizens' Panels – Conference on the Future of Europe'. Available at: https://futureu.europa.eu/en/pages/european-citizens-panels (accessed 19 July 2023).

Felt, U. and Fochler, M. (2010) 'Machineries for making publics: inscribing and de-scribing publics in public engagement', *Minerva*, 48(3): 219–238. https://doi.org/10.1007/s11024-010-9155-x

Ferguson, E. (2022) 'Sue Gray Partygate report: 59% of public think Boris Johnson should quit but just 7% think he will, poll finds', *The Independent*. Available at: https://inews.co.uk/news/politics/sue-gray-partygate-report-boris-johnson-resign-1650603 (accessed 19 July 2023).

Freedman, L. (2020) 'Scientific advice at a time of emergency. SAGE and Covid-19', *The Political Quarterly*, 91(3): 514–522. https://doi.org/10.1111/1467-923X.12885

G1000 (2022) 'Brussels launches world's first permanent Citizens' Assembly on Climate'. Available at: www.g1000.org/en/news/brussels-launches-worlds-first-permanent-citizens-assembly-climate (accessed 19 July 2023).

GOV.UK (2020) 'Prime Minister's statement on coronavirus (COVID-19): 18 March 2020'. Available at: www.gov.uk/government/speeches/pm-statement-on-coronavirus-18-march-2020 (accessed 19 July 2023).

GOV.UK (2021) 'Making vaccination a condition of deployment in older adult care homes'. Available at: www.gov.uk/government/consultations/making-vaccination-a-condition-of-deployment-in-older-adult-care-homes/making-vaccination-a-condition-of-deployment-in-older-adult-care-homes (accessed 19 July 2023).

GOV.UK (2022) 'Moral and Ethical Advisory Group'. Available at: www.gov.uk/government/groups/moral-and-ethical-advisory-group (accessed 19 July 2023).

Greubel, J. (2022) 'A new generation of European Citizens' Panels: making citizens' voices a regular part of policymaking', *European Policy Centre*. Available at: www.epc.eu/en/publications/A-new-generation-of-European-Citizens-Panels~4b959c (accessed 19 July 2023).

Helm, T. and Savage, M. (2023) 'Labour to omit funding of social care reform from manifesto and scale back Lords plans', *The Observer*. Available at: www.theguardian.com/politics/2023/oct/15/labour-to-omit-social-care-reform-from-manifesto-and-scale-back-lords-plans (accessed 7 December 2023).

Hopkins Van Mil (2021) 'Pandemic ethics: a public dialogue'. Available at: https://static1.squarespace.com/static/56f16de77da24f3e5612733b/t/614c8bae3d881c1e28957279/1632406454206/HVM+Pandemic+Ethics+Report+Sep21.pdf (accessed 19 July 2023).

Hopkins Van Mil (2023) 'Hopkins Van Mil'. Available at: http://www.hopkinsvanmil.co.uk (accessed 19 July 2023).

Involve (2022) 'Developing a Data Charter with residents'. Available at: www.involve.org.uk/resources/blog/news/developing-data-charter-residents (accessed 19 July 2023).

JCVI (2021) 'JCVI statement on COVID-19 vaccination of children aged 12 to 15 years: 3 September 2021', GOV.UK. Available at: www.gov.uk/government/publications/jcvi-statement-september-2021-covid-19-vaccination-of-children-aged-12-to-15-years/jcvi-statement-on-covid-19-vaccination-of-children-aged-12-to-15-years-3-september-2021 (accessed 19 July 2023).

Kirkpatrick, D. and Mueller, B. (2020) 'U.K. backs off medical rationing plan as coronavirus rages', *The New York Times*, 3 April. Available at: www.nytimes.com/2020/04/03/world/europe/britain-coronavirus-triage.html (accessed 19 July 2023).

Kuylen, M. et al. (2021) 'Should age matter in COVID-19 triage? A deliberative study', *Journal of Medical Ethics*, 47(5): 291–295. https://doi.org/10.1136/medethics-2020-107071

Landemore, H. (2013) 'Deliberation, cognitive diversity, and democratic inclusiveness: an epistemic argument for the random selection of representatives', *Synthese*, 190: 1209–1231. https://doi.org/10.1007/s11229-012-0062-6

Landemore, H. (2020) *Open Democracy: Reinventing Popular Rule for the Twenty-First Century*, Princeton, NJ: Princeton University Press. https://doi.org/10.2307/j.ctv10crczs

Landler, M. and Castle, S. (2020) 'The secretive group guiding the U.K. on coronavirus', *The New York Times*. Available at: www.nytimes.com/2020/04/23/world/europe/uk-coronavirus-sage-secret.html (accessed 19 July 2023).

Manku, K. (2022) 'Westminster workshop summary: building public values into pandemic recovery and preparedness', UK Pandemic Ethics Accelerator. Available at: https://ukpandemicethics.org/wp-content/uploads/2022/07/Ethics-Accelerator-Westminster-Workshop-summary.pdf (accessed 19 July 2023).

Marmot, Sir M. et al. (2020) 'Build back fairer: the COVID-19 Marmot Review', The Health Foundation. Available at: www.health.org.uk/publications/build-back-fairer-the-covid-19-marmot-review (accessed 19 July 2023).

Mason, R. and Brooks, L. (2022) 'Labour unveils plan to overhaul constitution and replace the Lords', *The Guardian*. Available at: www.theguardian.com/politics/2022/dec/04/labour-unveils-overhaul-constitution-replace-houes-of-lords (accessed 19 July 2023).

Mavron, N. (2021) 'Coronavirus and compliance with government guidance UK: April 2021', ONS. Available at: www.ons.gov.uk/peoplepopulationandcommunity/healthandsocialcare/conditionsanddiseases/bulletins/coronavirusandcompliancewithgovernmentguidanceuk/april2021 (accessed 19 July 2023).

Nabben, K. (2021) 'Hacking the pandemic: how Taiwan's digital democracy holds COVID-19 at bay', *The Conversation*. Available at: http://theconversation.com/hacking-the-pandemic-how-taiwans-digital-democracy-holds-covid-19-at-bay-145023 (accessed 19 July 2023).

OECD (2020) *Innovative Citizen Participation and New Democratic Institutions: Catching the Deliberative Wave*. Paris: Organisation for Economic Co-operation and Development. Available at: www.oecd-ilibrary.org/governance/innovative-citizen-participation-and-new-democratic-institutions_339306da-en (accessed 19 July 2023).

Oliver, D. (2021) 'David Oliver: What price the Nolan principles for public office holders?', *BMJ*, 373, n935. https://doi.org/10.1136/bmj.n935

ONS (2023) 'Coronavirus (COVID-19) – Office for National Statistics'. Available at: www.ons.gov.uk/peoplepopulationandcommunity/healthandsocialcare/conditionsanddiseases (accessed 19 July 2023).

Oswald, M. and Laverty, L. (2021) 'Data sharing in a pandemic: three Citizens' Juries', National Institute for Health Research. Available at: https://arc-gm.nihr.ac.uk/media/Resources/ARC/Digital%20Health/Citizen%20Juries/New%2012621_NIHR_Juries_Report_WEB.pdf (accessed 19 July 2023).

Participedia (2021a) 'Bristol Citizens' Assembly'. Available at: https://participedia.net/case/7218 (accessed 19 July 2023).

Participedia (2021b) 'Camden Health and Care Citizens' Assembly'. Available at: https://participedia.net/case/7429 (accessed 19 July 2023).
Participedia (2021c) 'Scottish crowdsourcing exercise 'Coronavirus (COVID-19): framework for decision making'. Available at: https://participedia.net/case/6667 (accessed 19 July 2023).
Participedia (2021d) 'Scottish Parliament Citizens' Panel on COVID-19'. Available at: https://participedia.net/case/7381 (accessed 19 July 2023).
PHE (2021) 'Coronavirus Resources – Coronavirus Resource centre'. Archived at: https://discovery.nationalarchives.gov.uk/details/r/C17359593 (accessed 19 July 2023).
Prainsack, B. and Buyx, A. (2017) *Solidarity in Biomedicine and Beyond*, Cambridge: Cambridge University Press (Cambridge Bioethics and Law). https://doi.org/10.1017/9781139696593
Ramamurthy, A. et al. (2022) 'Nursing narratives: racism and the pandemic', The Pandemic and Beyond. Available at: https://pandemicandbeyond.exeter.ac.uk/wp-content/uploads/2022/03/nn-report_final.pdf (accessed 19 July 2023).
Riley-Smith, B. and Knapton, S. (2022) 'Plan B restrictions to be scrapped as Boris Johnson plots fightback', *The Telegraph*. Available at: www.telegraph.co.uk/politics/2022/01/14/plan-b-restrictions-scrapped-boris-johnson-plots-fightback/ (accessed 19 July 2023).
Rogers, A. (2022) 'People in the real world don't care about Partygate, Mark Spencer claims', *HuffPost UK*. Available at: www.huffingtonpost.co.uk/entry/mark-spencer-downing-street-parties-boris-johnson_uk_6203ef49e4b02f4ed47c71ea (accessed 19 July 2023).
Serco Institute (2021) 'Vaccine Passports & UK Public Opinion'. Available at: www.sercoinstitute.com/news/2021/vaccine-passports-uk-public-opinion (accessed 19 July 2023).
Siddique, H. (2022) 'Use of "VIP lane" to award Covid PPE contracts unlawful, High Court rules', *The Guardian*. Available at: www.theguardian.com/politics/2022/jan/12/use-of-vip-lane-to-award-covid-ppe-contracts-unlawful-high-court-rules (accessed 19 July 2023).
Skinner, G. (2021) 'Majority of Britons support extending certain COVID-19 restrictions, but not forever', Ipsos. Available at: www.ipsos.com/en-uk/majority-britons-support-extending-certain-covid-19-restrictions-not-forever (accessed 19 July 2023).
Slape, J. (2022) 'The role of PPIE in enabling rapid and trustworthy access to regional health data to support COVID-19 vaccine research', HDR UK. Available at: www.hdruk.ac.uk/case-studies/the-role-of-ppie-in-enabling-rapid-and-trustworthy-access-to-regional-health-data-to-support-covid-19-vaccine-research/ (accessed 19 July 2023).
Solomon, S. and Abelson, J. (2012) 'Why and when should we use public deliberation?', *The Hastings Center Report*, 42(2): 17–20. https://doi.org/10.1002/hast.27
Sortition Foundation (2021) 'Paris creates a permanent Citizens' Council'. Available at: www.sortitionfoundation.org/paris_creates_permanent_citizens_council (accessed 19 July 2023).

Traverse (2021) 'VacciNation: exploring vaccine confidence with people from African, Bangladeshi, Caribbean and Pakistani backgrounds living in England'. Available at: https://traverse.ltd/recent-work/reports/vaccination-exploring-vaccine-confidence-people-african-bangladeshi-caribbean-and-pakistani-backgrounds-living-england (accessed 19 July 2023).

UKRI (2020) 'Get funding for ideas that address COVID-19'. Available at: www.ukri.org/opportunity/get-funding-for-ideas-that-address-covid-19/ (accessed 19 July 2023).

Webb, J. (2021a) 'Ethical analysis of Conservative MPs' opposition to Covid-19 certification', UK Pandemic Ethics Accelerator. Available at: https://ukpandemicethics.org/wp-content/uploads/2021/12/Ethical-analysis-of-Conservative-MPs-opposition-to-covid-19-certification-1.pdf (accessed 19 July 2023).

Webb, J. (2021b) 'Pandemic public engagement: an ethical analysis', UK Pandemic Ethics Accelerator. Available at: https://ukpandemicethics.org/wp-content/uploads/2021/09/Pandemic-Public-Engagement-An-Ethical-Analysis.pdf (accessed 19 July 2023).

Webb, J. (2022) 'Pandemic public engagement tracker', UK Pandemic Ethics Accelerator. Available at: https://ukpandemicethics.org/library/pandemic-public-engagement-tracker/ (accessed 19 July 2023).

Weible, C. et al. (2012) 'Understanding and influencing the policy process', *Policy Sciences*, 45(1): 1–21. https://doi.org/10.1007/s11077-011-9143-5

Wilkinson, D. et al. (2020) 'Which factors should be included in triage? An online survey of the attitudes of the UK general public to pandemic triage dilemmas', *BMJ Open*, 10(12): e045593. https://doi.org/10.1136/bmjopen-2020-045593

Williams, S. and Michie, S. (2022) 'Covid-19: one year on from "Freedom Day," what have we learnt?', *BMJ*, 378: o1803. https://doi.org/10.1136/bmj.o1803

Williams, S. et al. (2020) 'Public perceptions and experiences of social distancing and social isolation during the COVID-19 pandemic: a UK-based focus group study', *BMJ Open*, 10(7): e039334. https://doi.org/10.1136/bmjopen-2020-039334

Wingate, S. (2022) 'Nadine Dorries claims "coup" brought down Boris Johnson', *The Independent*. Available at: www.independent.co.uk/news/uk/politics/nadine-dorries-coup-boris-johnson-b2122959.html (accessed 19 July 2023).

7

From a crisis of confidence towards confidence in a crisis: what can we learn about the pandemic's impact on democracy?

Reema Patel

Introduction and roadmap

In this chapter, I argue that an emergency public health response is most effectively implemented when liberal democratic nation states recognise that their mandate to govern stems from their adherence to the core principles that underpin ideals and notions of democracy. There has been substantial critique of the way in which 'illiberal democracies' deployed measures justifiable during the pandemic to entrench authoritarian power. Drawing from case studies and the empirical, deliberative research of the Ada Lovelace Institute and the Bingham Centre for the Rule of Law, I show that the impact on the health of liberal democracies was also markedly damaging and profound.

Core principles, such as the rule of law, human rights and good governance principles, were systematically undermined and overlooked in numerous liberal democratic governments' COVID-19 response. The effect of this was, I argue, to undermine the quality, effectiveness and legitimacy of government intervention – at a time when the government most relied on the confidence of its people – contributing to the longer term erosion of the health of democracy itself. In particular, the citizen juries undertaken during the lockdown by the Ada Lovelace Institute and the Bingham Centre for the Rule of Law found that, despite the state of emergency implemented during the lockdown, people continued to expect good governance during the pandemic and did not readily accept that democracy itself could be paused (Patel, 2020a).

In future crises, democratic nation states need to create participatory infrastructures, adapted to enable real-time collective dialogue, that complement the blunt instruments of emergency decision-making and act as a check against the risks of executive power overreach through (in effect) 'pausing democracy' or placing democracy itself in 'lockdown'. Such participatory infrastructures would support the maintenance of the quality and health of democracy. In this chapter, by reference to six short inter-related discussions and four evidence-based case studies (both from the coronavirus pandemic and other public health crises), I will take the reader through my developing argument. In concluding, I suggest that our empirically tested citizen jury model, piloted and adapted specifically for emergency situations, could (and, I argue, *should*) be adopted by policymakers going forward.

Discussion 1: Democrats relied on the social contract in a crisis, but also eroded it

> I wish to be somebody, not nobody; a doer, deciding, not being decided for. ... I feel free to the degree that I believe this to be true, and enslaved to the degree that I am made to realise it is not. (Berlin, 1969)

The use of emergency powers (as set out in the Public Health Act 1984 and Coronavirus Act 2020) imposed as a direct result of the UK government's COVID-19 response undeniably, eroded most people's sense of agency – their natural desire to 'be somebody', and to be free (Berlin, 1969).

This generated widespread resistance from some members of the public, manifesting in outright rejection of particular governmental policies such as mask wearing, vaccine uptake and lockdown restrictions (Kleitman et al., 2021). While policymakers, scientists and researchers opted for the simplistic narrative of assuming these individuals were 'misinformed' or 'disinformed', many risked overlooking substantive differences of viewpoints, values and perceptions that needed to be understood and engaged with directly (Nuffield Council on Bioethics and Involve, 2020). The state of emergency also contributed towards a concern among some members of the public that they were being reduced to passive 'recipients' of government policy in the crisis rather than active co-creators of the crisis response.

However, while specific individuals expressed concerns about their individual rights and freedoms being compromised due to the pandemic, the majority of people in liberal democracies did comply to some great extent with policies designed to manoeuvre their societies out of the crisis. However, their compliance does not suggest that they necessarily agreed that all exercise of emergency power was proportionate or accepted that democracy itself was a luxury in the pandemic that needed to be paused for the greater good.

On the contrary, I argue that compliance reflects adherence to a different viewpoint about democracy, even in a crisis. Social contract democracy theorists, for instance, propose that true liberty can only emerge from active participation in a society that secures the wellbeing and rights of its citizens through the establishment of a social contract (Rousseau, 2004 [1762]). This notion of a social contract is therefore founded on the premise that, without the existence of government and governmental intervention, life would be 'nasty, brutish and short' (Hobbes, 2008 [1651]).

In a more contemporary context, the work of both Rousseau and Hobbes has been adapted by Rawls to indicate that the social contract grounds justice itself in a democratic society – recognising that the source of these principles of justice and equity are themselves necessarily social (Rawls, 1999 [1971]). As the pandemic and the responses worldwide from governments and their citizens illustrate, without the existence of democratic infrastructures and government intervention at all, life would have indeed been nasty, brutish and short or, at the very least, nastier, more brutish and shorter – COVID-19 was a very real threat that required a swift, broad brush and collective societal response to contain its spread. This is borne out by research into compliance that suggests the key factors facilitating compliance were first, a desire to reduce risk to oneself and one's family and friends and then, to a lesser extent, to the general public. Also of importance were a desire to return to normality, the availability of activities and technological means to contact family and friends, and the ability to work from home (Wright et al., 2022). It was this notion of democracy that citizens accepted. Rather than a pausing of democracy itself, people continued to expect good governance during the pandemic, as findings from numerous citizen juries undertaken during the lockdown demonstrated (Patel, 2020a).

On the whole, politicians and policymakers did not understand that this was expected of them during COVID-19. Politicians asked people to both consider others and the long term in acting to address the pandemic but did not demonstrate their own trustworthiness in navigating the crisis (Annweiler et al., 2021). In failing to reassure and persuade their citizens that they were committed to the protection of democratic rights and liberties in the long term, and thereby to justify the extraordinary measures that they needed to take, politicians and policymakers created a crisis of confidence rather than confidence in a crisis (Patel, 2020a). In short, policymakers did not recognise that they were both relying on *and* seeking to reconstitute the 'social contract' at a time of crisis and asking citizens actively to co-create the (worse) new deal.

Internationally, a Freedom House (2020) study found that democracy itself was weakened in eighty countries, including liberal democracies, due to the pandemic. Among the study's 398 global civil society survey respondents, 27 per cent reported government abuse of power as one of the three issues most affected by the coronavirus outbreak. Worldwide, officials and security services perpetrated violence against civilians, detained people without justification and overstepped their legal authority (Freedom House, 2020).

I argue, with reference to UK and US examples, that these actions had the long-term effect of undermining the legitimacy of governmental actions and, thus, confidence in government, at a time when it was most needed to generate buy-in and compliance. It also impacted on the likely effectiveness of their interventions.

Discussion 2: States of emergency

Despite the fact that ministers required democracy itself to operate with confidence and legitimacy from the public, politicians in liberal democratic states almost universally entrenched executive power through a variety of mechanisms. Emblematic of this were the 'states of emergency' declared worldwide, which enabled governments to deal swiftly with the emergency, but also had the effect of actively concentrating untrammelled executive power and contorting the democratic state into an 'Emergency State' by eroding fundamental democratic constitutional checks and balances (Wagner, 2022). This was a worldwide phenomenon – in Israel, for example, the judiciary was suspended, electronic surveillance and the tracking of patients was implemented, and parliament was shut down for four days (Wagner, 2022), leading to claims that emergency powers had been pushed to their limits.

Even particular day-to-day choices in the UK, such as parliamentary and council decisions to return to deliberating in person during the pandemic while social distancing and mask wearing were necessary, had the effect of undermining the quality of debate and discussion (White and Lilley, 2021). This, therefore, had the effect of corroding the very institutional frameworks and structures on which government demands for public compliance relied. Fukuyama, for instance, found that the factors responsible for successful pandemic responses were state capacity, social trust and leadership and that even those historic liberal democracies that lacked those features struggled in their response to the pandemic (Fukuyama, 2020).

Discussion 3: Abrogation of the rule of law

Lord Bingham defined the rule of law in its essence in the following way: '*all persons and authorities* within the state, whether public or private, should be bound by and entitled to the benefit of laws publicly and prospectively promulgated and publicly administered in the courts' (Bingham, 2011).

During the pandemic, governments found they needed to ask, and sometimes require, or enforce, people to give up their individual freedoms to realise societal freedoms – crucially to enable a successful navigation out of the pandemic for everyone. Challenges arose when people decided not to comply, particularly when the rules were ignored by the very individuals responsible for creating them, as the trip to Barnard Castle by policymaker Dominic Cummings served to illustrate.

The 'Cummings effect' significantly shaped how the public perceived government policymaking – surveys undertaken during lockdown show that confidence in the government stabilised and improved in the fortnight prior to Cummings' trip to Barnard Castle, but that confidence suddenly decreased further after that event (Fancourt et al., 2020). Subsequent public and societal anger about the Downing Street parties underline this point – there remained the clear expectation that the application of all laws to all persons should remain, without exception. The independent investigation led by Sue Gray into the civil service Downing Street parties held during lockdown rules found: 'At least some of the gatherings in question represent a serious failure to observe not just the high standards expected of those working at the heart of Government but also of the standards expected of the entire British population at the time' (Gray, 2022: 7).

Discussion 4: Surveillance technologies

Unique to the COVID-19 pandemic was the rapid acceleration of technologies and the onset of electronic surveillance worldwide. At the same time as policymakers recognised how technologies could help citizens extend their sense of agency in day-to-day life through enabling remote work, remote education, remote council meetings, and opportunities to share knowledge and learning digitally, by way of example; some other technologies were rapidly accelerated in ways that did the opposite – they sought to exercise some level of government control over, or power to influence and shape, the behaviour of citizens.[1]

In Singapore, for instance, a COVID-19 digital contact tracing app, TraceTogether, was being accessed by the police for criminal investigations, despite reassurances of privacy from ministers (Han, 2021). Privacy experts increasingly expressed concern that governments would accumulate more personal information, with a view to shaping and influencing their citizens, than was necessary or proportionate to respond to the public health crisis, and would otherwise use that information to contravene the principles of individual autonomy and freedoms.

Despite substantial concerns about democracy and rights in the context of their use, they relied deeply on the conception of the social contract for their use and uptake, thus creating a highly compromised and ambivalent approach to their use at the outset by both citizens and policymakers. Two case studies follow, by reference to which I exemplify these concerns.

Case study 1: NHS Test and Trace contact tracing app (UK)

The UK's digital contact tracing app was a mobile application developed by the UK government to assist in the identification and notification of individuals who may have come into contact with someone infected with COVID-19. The app used Bluetooth technology to detect when two app users were in close proximity to each other for an extended period of time. If one user later tested positive for COVID-19, the app would alert other users who had been in close contact with that person and provide guidance on what steps to take next. The app was launched in September 2020, after a prolonged development period and some controversy due to concerns expressed by privacy organisations. It was initially only available in England and Wales, with Scotland taking a distinct approach.

The Test and Trace app was problematic for a number of reasons. There was a fundamental concern about its effectiveness in identifying close contacts. In addition, there were concerns over privacy and data protection, a lack of transparency in the development process, the potential for misuse and commercialisation of data and accessibility for people with disabilities. Additionally, the app was initially centralised, meaning that data were stored on a central server rather than on users' devices, raising concerns about government surveillance. Following an initial trial on the Isle of Wight, the Information Commissioner's Office[2] undertook a Data Protection Impact Assessment, and indicated the lack of clarity about data collection gave rise to concerns that its collection was not proportionate (Civil Service World, 2020). Overall, these issues highlighted the need for a more democratic and transparent approach to the development and implementation of digital technologies for public health purposes.

The UK's National Audit Office (NAO) published a report in December 2020 on the government's approach to Test and Trace during the COVID-19 pandemic, including the digital contact tracing app. The report highlighted several issues and challenges, including the delayed launch of the app and the need to integrate it with the existing manual contact tracing system.

The NAO also raised concerns about the effectiveness of the app, noting comparatively low levels of uptake for the level of public investment that development of the app had necessitated, and identifying that it was unclear what impact the app had had on reducing the spread of COVID-19 in the UK. It concluded that 'for as long as compliance is low, the cost-effectiveness of [NHS Test & Trace]'s activities will inevitably remain in doubt' (National Audit Office, 2020).

An international review of similar apps, including in Australia (New South Wales) and in Switzerland, found that digital contact tracing itself is a complex public health intervention depending not just on the functioning of the technology but also on its adoption by its users and on its wider integration into the broader public health response system. Despite the fact that similar technologies were rolled out internationally, levels of uptake and confidence varied enormously, suggesting that social factors (trust and confidence) played a key role in enabling uptake.

The [Swiss] study found that 'the optimal implementation of a digital contact tracing app must account for the epidemic context and deal with acceptability, privacy, and the respect of civil liberties' (Poletto and Boëlle, 2022). I go a step further than this to suggest that where there was a lack of confidence more broadly in the government's pandemic response, there was a lack of uptake.

Case study 2: Vaccine passports (UK)

Vaccine passports are documents or digital certificates that provide proof of a person's vaccination status against a particular disease, such as COVID-19. The purpose of vaccine passports is to allow vaccinated individuals to show that they are protected against the disease, thereby reducing the risk of spreading the disease to others.

In navigating the pandemic, numerous governments and nation states mooted the development of digital health and vaccine certificates. This generated considerable societal debate and controversy. Individual rights concerns arose from the potential for vaccine passports to be used as a tool for government surveillance and control. There were concerns about the potential for these passports to be used to restrict individual freedoms, such as the freedom of movement, and to create a 'two-tier society' where those who are or choose to be vaccinated have greater freedoms and opportunities than those who are not.

Others expressed the concern that vaccine passports did not guarantee immunity from infection or reinfection, and thus that the implementation of the initiative may risk increasing the prevalence and spread of COVID-19 inadvertently (Ada Lovelace Institute, 2021).

Despite those concerns, digital vaccine passports were also contextualised by proponents and governments as *enabling* democratic freedoms – yet again, manifesting the ambivalent democratic positioning of policymakers in relation to their use of the technology. As well as using the technology to exert some level of influence or control over citizens' freedom of movement, arguments positioned the technology *itself* as mediating increased access to individual rights and freedoms.

For instance, vaccine passports were suggested as a way to enable increased individual freedoms (presenting an opportunity to emerge from lockdown while minimising risk or exposure through vaccine certification) – the Tony Blair Institute for Global Change described them as the 'ultimate exit strategy' (Tony Blair Institute for Global Change, 2021). They were proposed as a mechanism to facilitate the safe resumption of activities such as international travel, large-scale sporting events and attendance at bars, restaurants and hotels.

However, in reality, they were often used in implicitly coercive ways – for instance, they were mandatory for international travel and thus enjoyed success and uptake due to people's appetite for travel. However, appetite for their use in domestic contexts remained limited – in the UK they were initially required for some venues in all of the four nations but were later phased out (White and Lilley, 2021).

This followed the finding from the Public Affairs and Constitutional Committee that the government should abandon its 'unjustified plans' and that the government had 'failed to make the scientific case' for their use (Public Administration and Constitutional Affairs Committee, 2021).

Discussion 5: The undermining of democracy in turn undermined the quality of science and data

Beyond the day-to-day of the pandemic response, this ambivalence also manifested at a different level – the 'science-led' approach claimed by policymakers existed in tension with the practical constraints of resourcing and truly enabling a data-driven approach. This resulted in the critique that 'following the science' mantra often adopted by policymakers had the effect of transforming science into a 'fig-leaf' for decisions that were predominantly values-laden and political in nature (Wagner, 2022). The narrative of 'scientism' from the UK government served to mask the reality of decision-making in the pandemic: while it was important for the government to be guided by scientific advice, good judgement and interpretation of societal values were equally (some might argue more) important. This, in turn, required collective intelligence at a time when the power to make decisions was concentrated in the hands of comparatively few. As events in the UK illustrated, there was a need for both more principled approaches to governance and more principled approaches to *government itself*, particularly by the front benches.

One of these approaches is epistemological pluralism, which essentially means an acceptance that we can know and understand things in alternative ways. This, despite the increasing evidence that points to the value of epistemological pluralism, and the importance of 'self-consciously recogniz[ing] the limits of [one's own] epistemology ... and engag[ing] with other approaches without attempting to usurp them' (Beaumont and de Coning, 2022).

Policymakers struggled with the epistemological openness that marks the feature of democratic society – what Popper described as the 'open society' (Popper, 1945). In such a society, epistemological pluralism is able to thrive – there is the recognition that knowledge itself (particularly the approach to science and policymaking) *requires* pluralism to develop and advance rather than the proposition of a single viewpoint.

In their efforts to deliver clear and consistent messaging about what was required for compliance from citizens, policymakers found themselves at times masking the rationale for their decisions or presenting only a singular perspective on the data. In so doing, they delivered a simplified view of COVID-19 itself, rather than acknowledging that their work was founded on assumptions and itself subject to an ongoing process of continuous and rapid epistemological inquiry.

In illustrating the risks generated by such an approach I turn to two further case studies – one from the time of cholera in the nineteenth century, and one from the COVID-19 pandemic itself.

Case study 3: The pump handle and John Snow

There is a saying, incorrectly attributed to Mark Twain, that states, 'History never repeats itself but it rhymes'. We can look towards the nineteenth-century cholera outbreak in London's Soho to identify some 'rhyming patterns' that might inform politicians' and policymakers' often conflicted and ambivalent approaches to data use and evidence (and thus, to a genuinely 'open society') in times of crisis.

In 1854, Snow's use of a dot map to illustrate clusters of cholera cases around public water pumps, and of statistics to establish the connection between the quality of water sources and cholera outbreaks, led to a breakthrough in public health interventions – and, famously, the removal of the handle of a water pump in Broad Street.

Although John Snow had persuaded government officials to remove the handle of the water pump he had linked to cholera cases in Soho, his own explanation of the cause of cholera outbreaks – that it was a water-borne disease – was rejected for months. The Board of Health issued a report that said, 'We see no reason to adopt this belief' – prompting Snow to continue to gather data about cases of cholera, tracing them back to the pump.

Scientific orthodoxy at the time preferred the 'miasma' theory – that cholera was caused by the inhalation of vapours in the atmosphere – and it took considerable time for Snow's hypothesis to be taken seriously. In the meantime, people were falling ill and dying.

There can be a discrepancy between what the data say we *should* do, and what governments *want* to do – other short-term economic and political pressures push against the evidence base, compounding a natural resistance to change.

Furthermore, as the examples of both NHS digital contact tracing and vaccine passports illustrate, *how* the data is generated is of great significance and importance. Equally likely to be the site of political contestation is the purposes for which the data is used.

The John Snow Society, at its annual Pumphandle Lecture, commemorates, through a ceremonial removal and reattachment every year of a pump handle, the medical world's ongoing struggle against such forces (Patel, 2020c). This example illustrates the importance of both data and other types of knowledge in addressing the crisis.

Thus, epistemic pluralism, a core feature of an open and democratic society, is itself central to liberal and democratic states navigating their way out of the pandemic, saving lives and offering timely responses to public health emergencies.

However, Case study 4 uses a more contemporary point from the pandemic to illustrate a similarly ambiguous relationship with evidence and data that policymakers exhibited worldwide.

Case study 4: Johns Hopkins data dashboard (USA)

Despite their claim to be 'led by science', many actions by policymakers served to suggest otherwise. A key example of a real-time resource established in the early days of the pandemic was the aggregated database established by Johns Hopkins University – a web-based dashboard that mapped (very rapidly) the growth rate of incidences of COVID-19 deaths and recovery cases across the world. This source of data was vital for policymakers and researchers to understand and track the incidence of COVID-19 worldwide.

The Johns Hopkins data dashboard became essential for decision-makers as it enabled them to track the spread of the virus worldwide, with the university reporting that the dashboard was viewed more than 2.5 billion times and that more than 200 billion requests for data were received.

However, the dashboard encountered (over time) significant resistance, with a number of US federal agencies and states failing to share data in a timely fashion, or at all. It also encountered barriers when it came to the standardisation and consistency of data collection worldwide.

Ultimately, the dashboard closed, due to the lack of adequate participation from governments around the world to provide an accurate perspective on transmission (Torkington, 2023).

The Coronavirus Research Centre (CRC), which hosted the data dashboard, found that, from 2021, US states and counties began to consistently reduce the amount of publicly reported data, leading the CRC to discontinue hourly reporting for testing and vaccine data. Public reporting continued to decline from then onwards.

Meanwhile, the federal government significantly expanded its data tracking and reporting capacities (Donovan, 2023).

As these examples illustrate, despite claims of being 'science led', the behaviour of policymakers, when it came to access to and control of data about the pandemic, contributed towards concerns that the science was instead being led by politics. This contributed to widespread societal concern, in turn undermining the spirit of epistemological inquiry that characterises a genuinely democratic and open society, but also undermining the potential for the effective functioning of science at a time when this was crucial for the effectiveness of policymaking (Popper, 1945). Yet again, the task for policymakers was to interpret and apply the principles of epistemological openness to the context of the crisis – rather than to reach immediately for and adopt the 'closed' epistemological model. The lessons of history (the cholera outbreak) as well as the instance of the Johns Hopkins database serve to illustrate this point.

Discussion 6: Towards confidence in a crisis – where next?

As part of a UKRI COVID-19 rapid-response grant, I was a co-investigator on behalf of the Ada Lovelace Institute, with researchers from the University of Edinburgh and the Bingham Centre for the Rule of Law, exploring citizens' views and values in the UK through the use of citizen juries. Our participants (n = 50) were demographically sampled to represent the diversity of the UK population, while including a significant number of individuals from clinically vulnerable groups and disproportionately affected minorities (Bingham Centre for the Rule of Law, 2020). The group was purposively sampled with a broad distribution of age, gender, ethnicity and location (rural, market town and urban split), with slight overrepresentation of those who were asked to shield due to COVID-19 vulnerability in the pandemic, to ensure adequate representation of their perspectives. They were recruited by the agency People for Research to meet the pre-identified quota sample and remunerated for their time to contribute.

This project, at the intersection of law, ethics, citizen deliberation, public health and data science, aimed to develop a values-based framework to help understand and address the challenges posed by data-driven responses to public health emergencies and the need to build public trust.

The juries that deliberated as part of this work examined a range of data-driven technologies deployed in response to the pandemic, including digital contact tracing, vaccine passports to enable freedom of movement, and the use of the Shielded Patients List to identify those most vulnerable.

The two online citizen juries were held during summer 2021. Each jury deliberated for four consecutive days. The jury process combined short briefings by experts, followed by extensive deliberation within the jury group and a final presentation of preferred regulatory frameworks to policymakers from the NHS, UK government and devolved administrations.

Jurors met for two-and-a-half hours each day from Monday to Thursday in a single week, to hear presentations and take part in facilitated discussions in breakout groups. Each jury followed the same structure:

- Day 1: Jurors were introduced to the project, provided with an overview of data-driven technologies deployed in response to the pandemic, and given some initial provocations around challenges for the rule of law and good governance to aid their deliberations.
- Days 2–3: Jurors were given presentations about their chosen case studies – vaccine passports, risk-scoring algorithms and the General Practice Data for Planning and Research programme (GPDPR) – from experts who spoke either for or against each case study. Following these discussions, jurors discussed the

technologies in depth in their deliberations – articulating 'green lights', 'red lines' as well as conditions and safeguards relating to the technologies themselves.
- Day 4: Jurors reflected on all they had heard in the previous days and discussed conclusions across the technologies – developing and co-creating principles for good governance in emergencies.

The process aimed to identify areas where there were substantial points of disagreement, as well as consensus, crystallising their deliberations into a set of principles for good governance of the use of the technologies that were discussed.

The process provided a fascinating window on the extent to which good governance and the rule of law were considered important by members of the public, not only in the context of pandemic response measures but also in relation to other democratic developments in data-driven technologies that could be anticipated in future (Patel et al., 2022).

Importantly, through the method of deliberation itself, we aimed to reflect in the juries the ambivalence, nuance and the wide range of values and views held by citizens more broadly, both in terms of the restrictions on their lives during lockdowns and in the context of the use of rapidly developing technologies.

The deliberative process also challenged participants to work together, putting the ambivalent and wide-ranging views to work as a tool for developing each jury's own views on good governance in a crisis. Informed by these deliberations, the Ada Lovelace Institute synthesised the seven key principles required for good governance of technologies.

I suggest that these principles need not be constrained to the technologies themselves, but have wider relevance, even to inform how democratic states might best govern themselves to (more) successfully navigate similar crises in future. This would help address the gap in the literature at which this book is directed – an initial review indicating that, despite the breadth of literature reviewing the impact of the pandemic in retrospect, there is markedly limited research and work seeking to articulate good governance, particularly by understanding the views of citizens themselves.

Thus, the work of the Ada Lovelace Institute and the Bingham Centre for the Rule of Law represents a contribution, not just to the debate about the good governance of technologies, but more

What was the pandemic's impact on democracy? 165

broadly, to an understanding of good governance for a public health response to a pandemic, mediated by rapidly developing technologies. In Table 7.1 I have adapted these seven principles to suggest how they might inform successful public health emergency decision-making and governance more widely.

Table 7.1 Seven principles for successful public health emergency decision-making and governance

Principle	Significance for crisis decision-making
Transparency, communication and clarity	To support clear and consistent communication on the use of public health measures in a crisis
Accountability	To reinforce the importance of adherence to the rule of law from all parties, including government and policymakers themselves Ensuring appropriate checks and balances are in place
Equity, inclusivity and non-discrimination	To ensure that the use of public health measures does not exacerbate inequities within society, or create a two-tiered society
Protection of personal freedoms	To ensure that public health measures, so far as possible, should recognise and respect individual freedoms and rights
Proportionate and time-limited measures	To ensure that public health measures strike the appropriate balance between public health needs and risks to individuals and society – pandemic response measures designed explicitly for the crisis must not extend into post-pandemic data futures
Emergency preparedness and planning supports epistemic pluralism	To acknowledge that effective, accurate and responsibly managed data and other relevant evidence form the basis for preparedness, planning and crisis response measures
Trustworthiness	Organisations and governance structures implementing a public health or emergency measure must be trustworthy, and must act in demonstrably trustworthy ways

In addition, participants articulated numerous 'red lines' – clear boundaries that public health decision-makers ought not to overstep. Again, while these were initially generated for the use of technologies as a public health intervention, they can be extrapolated more widely for public health measures in general. The citizen juries' 'red lines' were:

- Public health measures should not create a two-tiered society that disproportionately discriminates against or disadvantages certain groups.
- Any measures exceptionally and temporarily accepted during the pandemic should not be extended into the future, after the pandemic ends.
- Public health measures should not be used to surveil, influence, profile or predict the behaviour of individuals.

Institutionalising deliberation at a time of crisis: a conclusion

The process of public deliberation piloted by the Bingham Centre for the Rule of Law and by the Ada Lovelace Institute (through the pandemic) itself illustrates the potential for governments to operate in a deliberative and democratic manner, even at a time of significant pressure and crisis.

At a time where executive decision-making is concentrated in the hands of very few, there are significant benefits to broadening out consideration of decision-making on issues as controversial or challenging as vaccine passports or contact tracing to a broader range of viewpoints. The 'mini public', adapted to convene rapidly, represents a practical and feasible way to do so (Patel, 2020b).

Our work demonstrates the feasibility of creating an open society that can operate in an epistemologically pluralist way, combining policy and science with citizen values and expertise. I suggest it points to the potential for developing a scalable, real-time, responsive model that would enable policymakers to embed the principles of a democratic dialogue and a more open society even (and maybe especially) at a time when policymaking risks 'closing' societies and thereby 'locking down' democracy.

It is no surprise then, that as we emerge from the pandemic structures – for instance, the sunset clauses that provide for the expiry of emergency legislation such as the Coronavirus Bill in the UK (Davis and Cowie, 2020) and the broader return to due parliamentary process – we are tracing a shift away from 'scientisation' towards a deliberative and 'participatory turn' in policymaking, with policymakers and scientists increasingly appreciating the value of turning to the experiences of diverse citizens to help shape and inform better science, and better policymaking (Krick et al., 2019).

Our citizen jury data suggest that, in preparation for future crises, it is crucial that democratic nation states reflect (honestly and transparently) on their recent experiences, learn from these 'online deliberative debate' models and adopt them to help shape increasingly participatory and deliberative infrastructures for democracy in a crisis. These models of deliberation have the potential to engage policymakers and scientists in dialogue with the public and to co-create a vision for a future in which we are all shaped by the pandemic, but seek, constructively, to move beyond it.

More broadly, this chapter has shown that the best course for liberal democratic states to chart in effectively implementing their public health responses is to recognise that their mandate to govern stems from their adherence to core rule of law, human rights and good governance principles. We have seen that these key tenets of democratic government *matter* in protecting and promoting legitimacy, compliance and broader societal support and consensus around key policy measures during a major public health emergency.

During the pandemic, governments succumbed to the strong temptation to overreach their powers through the blunt instrument of the emergency powers at their disposal. They sought to control, nudge and influence the public, and to impose control in a 'top-down' manner.

However, as the case studies discussed above illustrate, there is limited evidence to demonstrate that this approach is (in the long term) wholly effective in enabling a swift and effective response to crises. Indeed, we might conclude such an approach is largely *ineffective*, the tendency to 'overreach' contributing towards diminishing trust and confidence in policymakers during the pandemic.

Numerous public deliberation exercises in the pandemic (Patel et al., 2022) found that, while citizens are willing to accept that policymakers face unusual pressures and may need to resort to unprecedented mechanisms and powers at their disposal, they expect the broad overarching frameworks of rule of law, good governance, proportionality, democracy and human rights to remain in place – and for public health measures taken to be transparently and clearly justified. Democratic states depend on their democratic mandate, even in a crisis, and must actively engage their citizens in reshaping their social contract if they are to avoid crises of confidence and, instead, create confidence in a crisis.

Notes

1 I note here that even those technologies and platforms that are positioned as 'neutral' mediators or brokers of dialogue and discussion themselves had the potential to gather data without adequate transparency for the users of digital services. Here, in the context of the pandemic, technologies presented a privacy/agency trade-off throughout, some more prominently than others.
2 The Information Commissioner's Office is the UK's privacy regulator.

References

Ada Lovelace Institute (2021) 'What place should COVID-19 vaccine passports have in society?'. Available at: www.adalovelaceinstitute.org/report/covid-19-vaccine-passports/ (accessed 12 October 2023).

Annweiler, C. et al. (2021) 'Is a new COVID-19 social contract appropriate?', *The Lancet Public Health*, 6(6): e363. https://doi.org/10.1016/s2468-2667(21)00092-x

Beaumont, P. and de Coning, C. (2022) 'Coping with complexity: toward epistemological pluralism in climate-conflict scholarship', *International Studies Review*, 24(4): viac055. https://doi.org/10.1093/isr/viac055

Berlin, I. (1969) 'Two concepts of liberty', in I. Berlin, *Four Essays on Liberty*, Oxford: Oxford University Press. Available at: www.wiso.uni-hamburg.de/fileadmin/wiso_vwl/johannes/Ankuendigungen/Berlin_twoconceptsofliberty.pdf (accessed 9 May 2015).

Bingham, T. (2011) *The Rule of Law*, London: Penguin.

Bingham Centre for the Rule of Law (2020) 'The role of good governance and the rule of law in building public trust in data-driven responses to public health emergencies'. Available at: https://binghamcentre.biicl.org/projects/the-role-of-good-governance-and-the-rule-of-law-in-building-public-trust-in-data-driven-responses-to-public-health-emergencies (accessed 15 April 2023).

Chachko, E. and Shiner, A. (2020) 'Israel pushes its emergency powers to their limits', *The Regulatory Review*, 28 April. Available at: www.theregreview.org/2020/04/28/chachko-shinar-israel-pushes-emergency-powers-limits/ (accessed 15 April 2023).

Civil Service World (2020) 'ICO tells NHS to "collect minimum amount of personal data" as contact-tracing app starts trial', 6 May. Available at: www.civilserviceworld.com/professions/article/ico-tells-nhs-to-collect-minimum-amount-of-personal-data-as-contacttracing-app-starts-trial (accessed 10 May 2023).

Davis, F. and Cowie, G. (2020) 'Coronavirus Bill: What is the sunset clause provision?', House of Commons Library. Available at: https://commonslibrary.parliament.uk/coronavirus-bill-what-is-the-sunset-clause-provision/ (accessed 12 October 2023).

Donovan, D. (2023) 'Johns Hopkins winds down pioneering pandemic data tracking', *The Hub*, 10 February. Available at: https://hub.jhu.edu/2023/02/10/coronavirus-resource-center-ending-tracking/ (accessed 12 October 2023).

Fancourt, D., Steptoe, A. and Wright, L. (2020) 'The Cummings effect: politics, trust, and behaviours during the COVID-19 pandemic', *The Lancet*, 396(10249): 464–465. https://doi.org/10.1016/s0140-6736(20)31690-1

Freedom House (2020) 'Democracy under lockdown'. Available at: https://freedomhouse.org/report/special-report/2020/democracy-under-lockdown (accessed 12 October 2023).

Fukuyama, F. (2020) 'The pandemic and political order', *Foreign Affairs*, 9 June. Available at: www.foreignaffairs.com/articles/world/2020-06-09/pandemic-and-political-order?check_logged_in=1&utm_medium=promo_email&utm_source=lo_flows&utm_campaign=registered_user_welcome&utm_term=email_1&utm_content=20230415 (accessed 15 April 2023).

Gray, S. (2022) 'Findings of Second Permanent Secretary's investigation into alleged gatherings on government premises during covid restrictions'. Available at: https://assets.publishing.service.gov.uk/government/uploads/system/uploads/attachment_data/file/1078404/2022-05-25_FINAL_FINDINGS_OF_SECOND_PERMANENT_SECRETARY_INTO_ALLEGED_GATHERINGS.pdf (accessed 12 October 2023).

Han, K. (2021) 'Broken promises: how Singapore lost trust on contact tracing privacy', *MIT Technology Review*, 11 January. Available at: www.technologyreview.com/2021/01/11/1016004/singapore-tracetogether-contact-tracing-police/ (accessed 12 October 2023).

Hobbes, T. (2008 [1651]) *Leviathan* (ed. J. C. A. Gaskin), Oxford: Oxford University Press.

Kleitman, S. et al. (2021) 'To comply or not comply? A latent profile analysis of behaviours and attitudes during the COVID-19 pandemic', *PLoS ONE*, 16(7): e0255268. https://doi.org/10.1371/journal.pone.0255268

Krick, E., Christensen, J. and Holst, C. (2019) 'Between "scientization" and a "participatory turn": tracing shifts in the governance of policy advice', *Science and Public Policy*, 46(6): 927–939. https://doi.org/10.1093/scipol/scz040

NAO (National Audit Office) (2020) 'The government's approach to Test and Trace in England: interim report'. Available at: www.nao.org.uk/reports/the-governments-approach-to-test-and-trace-in-england-interim-report/ (accessed 12 October 2023).

Nuffield Council on Bioethics and Involve (2020) 'Call for greater transparency and public involvement in the UK', press release, 28 April. Available at: www.nuffieldbioethics.org/news/nuffield-council-and-involve-call-for-greater-transparency-and-public-involvement-in-uk-response-to-covid-19-pandemic (accessed 12 October 2023).

Patel, R. (2020a) 'Confidence in a crisis?', Ada Lovelace Institute. Available at: www.adalovelaceinstitute.org/report/confidence-in-crisis-building-public-trust-contact-tracing-app (accessed 12 October 2023).

Patel, R. (2020b) 'Rapid, online deliberation on COVID-19 technologies', Ada Lovelace Institute. Available at: www.adalovelaceinstitute.org/project/rapid-online-deliberation-on-covid-19-technologies/ (accessed 14 April 2023).

Patel, R. (2020c) 'Removing the pump handle: stewarding data at times of public health emergency', *Significance Magazine*, 20 May. Available at: https://significancemagazine.com/removing-the-pump-handle-stewarding-data-at-times-of-public-health-emergency/ (accessed 15 April 2023).

Patel, R., Peppin, A. and Machirori, M. (2022) 'The rule of trust', Ada Lovelace Institute. Available at: www.adalovelaceinstitute.org/wp-content/uploads/2022/07/The-rule-of-trust-Ada-Lovelace-Institute-July-2022.pdf (accessed 15 April 2023).

Poletto, C. and Boëlle, P.-Y. (2022) 'Learning from the initial deployment of digital contact tracing apps', *The Lancet Public Health*, 7(3): 206–207. https://doi.org/10.1016/S2468-2667(22)00035-4

Popper, K. (1945) *The Open Society and Its Enemies*, London: Routledge.

Public Administration and Constitutional Affairs Committee (2021) 'No justification for COVID passports say committee'. Available at: https://committees.parliament.uk/committee/327/public-administration-and-constitutional-affairs-committee/news/155788/no-justification-for-covid-passports-say-committee/ (accessed 12 October 2023).

Rawls, J. (1999 [1971]) *A Theory of Justice* (rev. edn), Cambridge, MA: Harvard University Press.

Rousseau, J.-J (2004 [1762]) *The Social Contract* (trans. M. Cranston), London: Penguin.

Tony Blair Institute for Global Change (2021) 'The UK Government should take the lead on implementing digital health passports – here's why', Commentary 14 February. Available at: www.institute.global/insights/public-services/uk-government-should-take-lead-implementing-digital-health-passports-heres-why (accessed 12 December 2023).

Torkington, S. (2023) 'The world's leading COVID-19 tracker is closing down – here's why', *World Economic Forum*, 9 March. Available at: www.weforum.org/agenda/2023/03/covid-tracker-closing-down-johns-hopkins/ (accessed 12 October 2023).

Wagner, A. (2022) *Emergency State*, London: Bodley Head.

White, H. and Lilley, A. (2021) 'Parliament's role in the coronavirus crisis: holding the government to account', Institute for Government, 27 May. Available at: www.instituteforgovernment.org.uk/publication/parliaments-role-coronavirus-crisis (accessed 15 April 2023).

Wright, L. et al. (2022) 'Facilitators and barriers to compliance with COVID-19 guidelines: a structural topic modelling analysis of free-text data from 17,500 UK adults', *BMC Public Health*, 22, article 34. https://doi.org/10.1186/s12889-021-12372-6

8

Accountability, transparency and good governance: the WHO's decision-making during an emergency

Harry Upton, Abbie-Rose Hampton and Mark Eccleston-Turner

The World Health Organization (WHO) has a broad, expansive role during a health emergency, and despite the proliferation of NGOs and public-private partnerships into global health in the past twenty years (Anbazhagan and Surekha, 2021), as well as other international actors encroaching upon the WHO's mandate (Burci, 2014), it remains the central actor in global health governance. Traditionally, the role of the WHO has been normative in nature, providing advice and guidance to member states on best practice during a health emergency. Indeed, the Organization historically viewed itself as merely a norm-setting body, gathering scientific evidence, synthesising it, and communicating it to member states, and, increasingly, to the general public. However, this role shifted significantly in 2003 during, and after, the outbreak of severe acute respiratory syndrome (SARS), a viral respiratory disease caused by a SARS-associated coronavirus. The WHO director-general at this time took unprecedented steps to recommend travel restrictions to mitigate spread of the virus, including direct calls to action aimed at private industry as well as governments (Eccleston-Turner and Wenham, 2021). Throughout the SARS outbreak, the WHO became central to collating and analysing data, providing technical guidance to states, and indeed travel and trade recommendations to minimise the disease's spread, even when it had no explicit legal mandate to do so (Heymann and Roider, 2004; Kamradt-Scott, 2010). Indeed, as Kamradt-Scott observed, the WHO now found itself acting simultaneously as 'real time epidemic coordinator, policy advisor, government assessor, and government critic' (Kamradt-Scott, 2015). Such was the perceived success of this new role for the organisation during SARS that this role was 'legalised' through the post-SARS reforms to the International Health Regulations (IHR) in 2005 (WHO, 2005), where 'the alert and response mechanisms of the [revised] IHR are modelled on the tools, processes and assumptions that characterized the global response to SARS' (Burci and Eccleston-Turner, 2020).

Despite the fact that the IHR – the singular piece of binding international law governing infectious disease outbreaks – is intended to 'prevent, detect against, control, and provide a public health response to'[1] the spread of infectious diseases, it is overly focused on prevention and detection, and plays a very limited role in the direct response to an outbreak, beyond affording the director-general the power to make recommendations, in highly limited, specific circumstances (Eccleston-Turner, 2023), recommendations which are often ignored by member states, who prioritise their own self-interest in response to an infectious disease outbreak, rather than the collective good (Tejpar and Hoffman, 2017; Mason Meier et al., 2022). Despite this rather limited explicit legal mandate, the WHO does carry out a number of response functions during a health emergency that go beyond the normative. Most notably, the WHO is actively involved in the procurement and delivery of medical supplies, such as through the COVAX Facility during COVID-19 and the WHO Pandemic Influenza Preparedness Framework, attempting to counter the huge global injustice in access to medicines which exists during health emergencies (Eccleston-Turner and Upton, 2021a, 2021b; Hampton et al., 2021). In some circumstances, such as Ebola in West Africa and the recent outbreaks in the Democratic Republic of the Congo, the WHO has gone as far as to provide health services in a 'boots on the ground' manner (Gostin and Friedman, 2014; Wenham, 2017). Due to the limitations of the legal structure of the IHR, these vital response activities are not grounded in IHR, but rather done on the basis of the constitutional mandate of the director-general.

The fact that these operational activities exist outside the legal framework for health emergencies provided by the IHR gives rise to some important questions about accountability and good governance, particularly when things go wrong, or the operations do not function as intended. This chapter begins by outlining why good governance matters for international organisations, notably good governance as a 'soft' legal concept, as well as a hard one; it then goes on to question the binary nature of an 'emergency' and 'non-emergency' distinction, upon which much of the discussions on this issue have been predicated to date; and finally, considers the governance of the WHO's operational activities during a health emergency.

Why good governance matters

The COVID-19 pandemic has served as the most recent reminder that while good global health governance (GHG) is understood to be vital for an effective and efficient coordinated response to emerging health threats on a global scale (Gostin et al., 2020), the current system ultimately lacks the means and mechanisms through which to ensure good GHG within and between key organisations in global health, most notably the WHO. From the WHO's initial response to the emergence of COVID-19 – which was criticised by many as being 'inordinately slow' (Larinova and Kirton, 2020: 13) – to the organisation's participation in COVAX amid mounting pressure to achieve global vaccine equity – with the WHO's authority and calls for solidarity being ignored in favour of policies aligned with vaccine nationalism (Gostin et al., 2020) – the COVID-19 pandemic has marked a new wave of concern with regards to the level of trust in the WHO and the organisation's legitimacy overall as the central actor in GHG. The criticism surrounding the WHO's COVID-19 response has sparked discussions and debate with regards to the reimagining of GHG in a post-COVID world (Gostin et al., 2020: Larinova and Kirton, 2020), with it being clear that the achievement of good GHG is vital to rebuild trust in the organisation, although there is considerably less consensus as to what that would involve in practice.

While GHG is understood to be something of a 'slippery' concept (Lee and Kamradt-Scott, 2014: 5), with an array of definitions existing within the literature, it is broadly understood to refer to the framework of principles, arrangements, norms and processes (Lisk and Šehović, 2020: 48) utilised by the multitude of actors who share responsibility for addressing and responding to issues in global health (Eccleston-Turner et al., 2018). The actors involved here range from state and non-state actors to international organisations; with the WHO's role in GHG (WHO, 2013) relating directly to the powers and responsibility conferred upon it in its Constitution to act as 'the directing and coordinating authority on international health work' (WHO, 1948: Article 2(a)). Pressure is mounting, however, as a result of the growing need to achieve 'good' GHG (Eccleston-Turner and Villarreal, 2022). Precisely what constitutes good GHG, alongside its purpose, has been the subject of much debate within academic and policy circles but, despite the lack of clarity around its precise meaning, its achievement is a clear expectation for all actors involved with GHG (Lee and Kamradt-Scott, 2014); good governance appears to fall into the category of concepts which are difficult to define, but 'I know it when I see it', a quote made famous by the US Supreme Court decision in *Jacobellis v. Ohio*.[2] While variations of the key indicators do exist, the principles of transparency and accountability remain consistent as the twin tenets of good GHG (Buse and Walt, 2002) with additional indicators including legitimacy, effectiveness and respect for the rule of law (Lee and Kamradt-Scott, 2014).

The need for greater transparency forms the starting point in the bid to achieve good GHG, with its centrality being widely recognised by academics and policymakers alike (Storey and Eccleston-Turner, 2022). While transparency has 'no fixed meaning' and its features are open to interpretation (Gostin and Mok, 2009), the need for transparency in 'the decision-making process and the implementation of ... decisions', as well as 'access to information open to all potentially concerned and/or affected by the decisions at stake' (Storey and Eccleston-Turner, 2022), is vital at both the national and international level. While much of importance attributed to transparency in the context of good GHG emerges as a result of it amounting to an 'enforcement mechanism' which can be seen to facilitate or ensure the accountability of GHG institutions, of equal importance is its ability to produce trust and legitimacy (Storey and Eccleston-Turner, 2022). In taking the necessary steps to ensure transparency with regards to the processes and practices utilised by the varying institutions, the relevant stakeholders – such as WHO member states, and increasingly during COVID-19, the general public – are able to develop a clear understanding of how and why decisions have been made, with this often leading to the production of confidence or trust in these practices and, if not, placing stakeholders in a position to call for change and improvements (Storey and Eccleston-Turner, 2022).

Thus, a potential consequence of a lack of transparency at the WHO is reduced trust in the organisation from member states. The result of this is likely to be a lack of willingness to follow WHO recommendations during times of emergency, ultimately causing further damage to its reputation. An example of this can be seen with the widespread use of travel restrictions in the early stages of the COVID-19 pandemic. By April 2020, ninety-six countries had imposed travel restrictions or blanket bans on travel to and from China, where the outbreak was first identified, and approximately 90 per cent of commercial air traffic was grounded, following the introduction of global travel restrictions by 130 countries (Devi, 2020; Kiernan et al., 2020). These restrictions were introduced contrary to the Temporary Recommendations that had been issued by the WHO director-general, following the advice of the IHR Emergency Committee Regarding the Coronavirus Disease Pandemic, which called for states to avoid the introduction of travel restrictions at that time (WHO, 2020; COVID-19 IHR Emergency Committee, no date). This led some scholars to suggest that states had breached their obligations under Article 43 of the IHR, calling into question the ability of the WHO to command the confidence of its member states during an emergency (Habibi et al., 2020; Meier et al., 2020).

As for accountability, while this again has a variety of definitions, it is typically understood to ensure the acceptance of responsibility for one's actions, alongside the provision of both explanations and justifications (Eccleston-Turner et al., 2018). It is 'fundamental to the exercise of power', with GHG actors being expected to have comprehensive mechanisms in place which facilitate the scrutiny of processes, decisions and the subsequent consequences (Eccleston-Turner et al., 2018). For the most part, accountability is therefore largely concerned with the obligations of an institution (Eccleston-Turner et al., 2018), particularly with regards to whether they have been carried out in a satisfactory manner, and to account for the decision or failure to exercise relevant powers (Eccleston-Turner and McArdle, 2017). While accountability may seem like a relatively simple concept to understand, its implementation typically produces difficulties, taking place across multiple levels and incorporating a vast number of requirements (Eccleston-Turner and McArdle, 2017). What is clear, however, is that accountability mechanisms must ensure that GHG institutions are held to account for their actions as much as they hold others accountable, while going beyond purely internal accountability to include external accountability also (Eccleston-Turner and McArdle, 2017). Engaging with the concept of accountability and implementing comprehensive accountability mechanisms is, therefore, vital for good GHG; with the decisions made by GHG institutions often meaning the difference between life and death for the populations of affected nations, particularly during the exercise of emergency powers. External stakeholders must be able to demand explanations and justifications for actions which undermine their national interests or put the lives of their populations at risk but mechanisms which facilitate both transparency (Gostin and Mok, 2009) and accountability are severely lacking at the international level.

Despite the vast responsibilities and powers afforded to the WHO by both its Constitution and the IHR (WHO, 2005), the legitimacy of the organisation has ultimately been called into question as a result of a lack of transparency and the failure to implement comprehensive accountability mechanisms, which are sufficiently robust to defend the organisation from external critique (Eccleston-Turner and McArdle, 2020). COVID-19 has clearly highlighted the tensions which exist in times of emergency between the desires of the WHO to respond effectively and promptly to a health emergency, and the need to pursue transparency and accountability. Indeed, the very fact that an event is an emergency has been used to minimise the importance of accountability and checks and balances or sidestep them entirely.[3] Therefore, greater consideration must be afforded to the different modes of accountability utilised both within and beyond the organisation in a bid to ensure the achievement of good GHG, even during an emergency event.

A 'legal' emergency

For the most part when considering the good governance of the WHO in an emergency, the focus is on the formal, legal structures the WHO uses to operate during an emergency, that is, the IHR

(WHO, 2005). The IHR is the singular binding international legal instrument governing global health security, and central to the activities of the WHO within the regulations is the declaration of a public health emergency of international concern (PHEIC). A PHEIC declaration is made by the WHO director-general, on advice of the Emergency Committee, and empowers the director-general to make Temporary Recommendations to states that, while non-binding, seek to provide public health guidance and counteract unnecessary restrictions states may seek to place on international trade and travel (WHO, 2005; Art. 15). In addition, the PHEIC is typically seen as a clarion call to the international community (Gostin et al., 2019) that there is an outbreak on the horizon, but crucially fails to allocate the WHO or states additional financing in order to prepare and respond. A PHEIC declaration, by its very nature aligned with states of emergency elsewhere in governance structures, can bring the outbreak to the attention of governments beyond the health portfolio, including at presidential or cabinet level, and importantly into the treasury and/or department of defence, mobilising financial and technical assistance (Eccleston-Turner and Wenham, 2021). Indeed, the purported impact of a PHEIC declaration is one of the compelling reasons for its declaration (Gostin et al., 2019). Much has been written about governance of PHEICs, and the explicit powers they confer upon the WHO to act in an emergency (see, for example, Fidler, 2005; Fidler and Gostin, 2006; Eccleston-Turner and Wenham, 2021; Wenham et al., 2021), as well as the need for good governance of these emergency powers, and the accountability and control mechanism surrounding the use of explicit legal powers in a health emergency by the WHO (Eccleston-Turner and Wenham, 2021; Eccleston-Turner and Villarreal, 2022). However, this only tells part of the story, and there are a number of instances where the WHO operationally acts during an emergency, but does so beyond the confines of the PHEIC and the governance system created by the regulations.

For example, there are a number of instances whereby a PHEIC declaration is not made, but the WHO still becomes operationally involved in the response. One such case was the 2014 outbreak of Ebola in West Africa, when the WHO deployed epidemiologists there, and established initial contact tracing, laboratory support and infection control mechanisms, mirroring that which they had implemented in previous Ebola outbreaks (Wenham, 2017), despite the fact that an Emergency Committee had at that point not even met to consider declaring the event a PHEIC. Moreover, during the 2018 Ebola outbreak, the WHO consistently refused to declare the event a PHEIC (despite it being clear the criteria were met (Eccleston-Turner and Wenham, 2021)). By contrast, the WHO was still issuing advice to member states about the application of international travel or trade restrictions, stating that 'the Committee does not consider entry screening at airports or other ports of entry to be necessary' (WHO, no date). While this advice is similar to the content of many formal recommendations issued previously under the IHR, it was not promulgated in accordance with the procedure laid out in the regulations, meaning the recommendations lacked normative force and a legitimate basis in the legal structures for health emergency response. Indeed, there are numerous instances where a declaration of a PHEIC has not been made, or has been delayed for wider political reasons, yet the WHO responds to these emergency events (in a normative and operational manner). In such instances the organisation responds outside of the confines of the legal structures and processes created in the regulations for health emergency response. Further, as the following section lays out, the WHO has an entire programme of work on emergency response, which is not structurally aligned to the IHR or the declaration of a PHEIC, in that, the WHO Health Emergencies (WHE) Programme does not require a PHEIC declaration to trigger its activities.

Moving beyond the legal emergencies: WHO Health Emergencies Programme and COVAX

WHO Health Emergencies (WHE) Programme

The WHO Health Emergencies (WHE) Programme was established in 2016 following the Ebola epidemic in West Africa. The WHE Programme was designed to consolidate all of the WHO's work during health emergencies into a single programme, creating a common structure across all regional offices in order to increase efficiency and cooperation during health emergencies (United Nations (UN), 2016). The programme was designed: 'to bring speed and predictability to WHO's emergency work, using an all-hazards approach, promoting collective action, and encompassing preparedness, readiness, response and early recovery activities' (UN, 2016; para. 10). As part of the WHE Programme, the WHO aims to initiate an on-the-ground assessment within seventy-two hours of being notified of a high-threat pathogen, clusters of unexplained deaths in low-capacity settings or any other event to be determined at the discretion of the director-general (UN, 2016). The programme is headed by an executive director, but ultimately authority for the WHO's work in emergencies remains with the director-general.

The WHE Programme is overseen by the Independent Oversight and Advisory Committee (IOAC), which was established to provide independent scrutiny of the WHO's work during emergencies, following organisational and operational failings during the response to the West Africa Ebola epidemic. The first report of the IOAC urged the WHO 'to undertake major transformation in order to strengthen its organisational capacity to respond to outbreaks and other emergencies, and to restore trust and confidence in its ability to protect global health' (UN, 2020).

While the WHE Programme has sought to address the shortcomings of the response to Ebola in West Africa, the IOAC has raised several ongoing issues that must urgently be addressed to ensure that the programme functions to the best of its abilities. One such issue is capacity; the report of the IOAC to the 74th World Health Assembly revealed that the WHE Programme is 'inadequately equipped to deal with a global pandemic while simultaneously responding to other emergencies' (Syam and Alas, 2021). This issue with capacity is linked to what the IOAC called 'chronic underfunding' (UN, 2020), but also to concerns surrounding the ability of the programme to recruit, retain and manage an appropriately skilled workforce to support the work of the programme during emergencies (UN, 2020). Furthermore, while the WHE Programme has successfully engaged in partnerships with civil society and the private sector, such as the Access to COVID-19 Tools (ACT) Accelerator, urgent work is need to clarify the governance structure of WHO partnerships, including ensuring greater transparency at all levels (UN, 2020).

While the introduction of the WHE Programme may have improved communication within the wider WHO structure, it falls short of introducing the kind of structural changes needed to

Accountability, transparency, good governance 181

effect significant change to governance within the organisation. For example, the common structure of the WHE Programme has been relied upon to improve coordination between the WHO's regional offices, but some have suggested that use of the programme in this way simply masks the need for more comprehensive governance reforms, including restructuring of the regional offices, and therefore represents a 'governance drift' rather than a much-needed 'governance shift' (Mackey, 2016). There is also concern from some commentators that the WHE Programme may weaken the norm-setting function of the WHO by drawing precious resources into functions and operations associated with 'permanent firefighting' (Yach, 2016).

Such concerns surrounding the governance of the WHO, particularly with regards to accountability and transparency within the organisation or rather the lack thereof, are further exacerbated in the instances whereby the WHO operates through an external Public-Private-Partnership (PPP). Most recently, this has been evidenced during the COVID-19 pandemic through the WHO's participation in COVAX, with the remainder of this section offering an insight into the varying issues, questions and concerns surrounding the governance of the organisation which have emerged as a result.

COVAX

Throughout the COVID-19 pandemic, the WHO has acted as one of the main partner organisations of COVAX, the global, multilateral initiative designed to secure equitable access to COVID-19 vaccines (Eccleston-Turner and Upton, 2021a). Its participation raises some interesting questions about accountability at the WHO during its participation in extraordinary partnerships such as COVAX and the COVAX Facility.

For example, one relevant enquiry is to ask whether the WHO's involvement in the COVAX Facility's procurement of vaccines is compatible with the WHO's responsibility to be accountable to its member states. This issue is somewhat complicated by the confidential nature of COVAX's advance purchase agreements (APAs) and the involvement of other actors, such as Gavi the Vaccine Alliance and The Coalition for Epidemic Preparedness Innovation (CEPI), in their negotiation and completion. Like APAs conducted by the governments of individual states, the details of the purchase agreements completed on behalf of COVAX are generally confidential. This makes it difficult to understand the precise terms of the agreements reached by COVAX, with only details such as the total number of doses generally being made public. This complicates the assessment of the relative success that COVAX has had in negotiating its APAs compared to individual states, which in turn obstructs any inquiry into how well each of the partner organisations has been operating in terms of negotiating agreements for vaccine procurement (Hampton et al., 2021). In the context of vaccine procurement via COVAX, this is perhaps more of an issue for accountability at Gavi than it is for the WHO, because Gavi bears primary responsibility for negotiating purchase agreements on behalf of COVAX (Gavi, 2020). Nevertheless, the WHO is one of COVAX's main partner organisations. The fact that the precise details of what is perhaps the most important output of COVAX's work, the APAs, remains confidential is therefore a concern from the perspective of ultimate accountability to WHO member states.

Another question pertinent to the WHO's involvement in COVAX is how its engagement with the management and delivery of COVAX-supplied doses affects the WHO's obligations to its member states. Perhaps the WHO's main role in COVAX has been to coordinate and facilitate the delivery of the vaccines that COVAX has supplied, as well as additional doses donated by individual states. This has involved the creation of the WHO's 'Fair Allocation Framework', designed to ensure that the doses purchased by COVAX are split equitably between all of COVAX's participating economies (Eccleston-Turner and Upton, 2021a). In this context, 'equitable' distribution meant that doses were allocated so that countries received a similar number of doses relative to their population, although many high-income states chose to defer their early allocations, allowing more doses to be allocated to other participating states. In some ways, this aspect of the WHO's role in COVAX might be seen as being a practical way of fulfilling its mandate to promote the highest attainable standard of health among individuals within its member states. While COVAX has ultimately fallen short of its initial targets for vaccine delivery, it has nevertheless succeeded in delivering doses to participating states more quickly and in larger quantities than would have been possible if states had been left to fight entirely among themselves (Berkley, 2021). The WHO's role in leading the coordination of the delivery and utilisation of COVAX-supplied doses may therefore be seen as a way of the WHO fulfilling its constitutional mandate.

The question, in terms of accountability, is whether COVAX was the most appropriate mechanism through which the WHO could have pursued equitable access to vaccines. On the one hand, as referenced above, COVAX has contributed to improved, albeit not *equitable*, access to vaccines, particularly in low-income countries.[4] However, on the other hand, the WHO should be accountable to *all* of its member states, not just those represented by COVAX. Furthermore, the WHO was just one of the partner organisations responsible for the operation of COVAX. This makes the lack of transparency regarding things such as the details of APAs conducted by Gavi more problematic from the perspective of accountability because, while Gavi was the primary negotiator for those deals, they are nevertheless part of the COVAX programme of which the WHO is a key partner. The question is whether or not these transparency concerns are outweighed by the benefits of the WHO's participation in COVAX.

This may be said to depend on whether or not the WHO could have done more to contribute to equitable access *outside* of the COVAX initiative. This is a difficult question to answer, but one way of doing so is to compare the deployment of COVAX vaccines to the delivery of vaccines to countries supported by the WHO's Vaccine Deployment Initiative (VDI) during the 2009-H1N1 influenza pandemic. The VDI was designed by the WHO to facilitate the donation of influenza vaccines from high-income countries with excess doses, to the low-income countries which had been unable to procure their own doses (WHO, 2011). It delivered a total of 78 million doses to low-income countries, out of 122 million doses which had been pledged by high-income donors (Eccleston-Turner and Upton, 2021b). The first of these doses arrived in recipient countries four months after vaccination campaigns got under way in high-income countries which had procured their own doses (Partridge and Kieny, 2010). By comparison, COVAX delivered its first doses to Ghana in 24 February 2021 (WHO, 2021) around two months after the first dose was administered in the UK (GOV. UK, 2021). In total, COVAX has now delivered more than 1 billion doses of vaccine (Gavi, no date). Thus, while COVAX has failed to meet its own targets, its contribution to equitable access to vaccines has arguably been greater than the VDI's was during the 2009-H1N1 pandemic. Naturally, it is impossible to know how the WHO would have fared had it operated a similar system on its own for COVID-19. However, the fact that COVAX has been more successful than the VDI, for which the WHO acted largely alone, suggests that the WHO's involvement with it was ultimately of benefit to its member states.

Conclusion

The role of the WHO during a health emergency has been described as 'managerial'. The use of emergency powers by this international organisation, therefore, has necessitated a consideration of the extent to which the use of these powers aligns with principles of good governance. To date, consideration of the WHOs emergency powers has been limited, in that they have focused on the *legal basis* of these powers, and the extent to which the exercise of emergency powers aligns with the powers, duties and obligations of the WHO as outlined in the IHR and the WHO Constitution. To this extent, the current debates are grounded within the ideas of responsibility for internationally wrongful acts – formal international law. Such considerations have been rather limited, largely because of the limited development of the law of responsibility for international organisations, and the fact that the rules and principles contained within it lack practical application, especially during an emergency (Eccleston-Turner and McArdle, 2020).

The present chapter has moved beyond this limited, wholly legal consideration of WHO emergency powers, by considering to what extent WHO actions in an emergency – beyond the formal legalistic approaches – are grounded in principles of good governance. Such a consideration is notable because accountability, transparency and good governance are inherently linked to trust and legitimacy; given the significant challenges to the epistemic authority of the WHO during the COVID-19 pandemic, activities which enhance the legitimacy of the organisation are of vital importance. Through an examination of the WHE and COVAX initiatives, and the WHO's involvement in them, the present chapter has demonstrated that there are very limited control mechanisms over the WHO during a health emergency. This is particularly apparent when the WHO operates through an external PPP such as COVAX, with this ultimately functioning to produce an additional layer of complexity with regards to the achievement of good governance. While concerns surrounding the levels of accountability, transparency and legitimacy within the WHO are by no means a new phenomenon – with trust in the organisation having somewhat declined over time as a result – the experiences throughout the COVID-19 pandemic have ultimately strengthened the need for *soft* forms of accountability and control over the WHO, especially during an emergency.

Notes

1 Article 2, IHR.
2 Justice Stewart, in attempting to define obscene publications famously quoted, 'I shall not today attempt further to define the kinds of material I understand to be embraced within that shorthand description ["hard-core pornography"], and perhaps I could never succeed in intelligibly doing so. But *I know it when I see it*, [emphasis added] and the motion picture involved in this case is not that.' *Jacobellis v. Ohio*, 378 U.S. 184 (1964), at 197.
3 At the international level see Eccleston-Turner and Villarreal, 2022. For a national perspective on emergency declarations being used to sidestep checks and balances see Grogan, 2022.
4 While 'equity' is difficult to define, the contention that COVAX has not delivered equitable access to vaccines is repeated here on the basis that (i) COVAX failed to meet its own target of delivering 2 billion doses before the end of 2021 and, as of April 2023, COVAX has still delivered fewer than 2 billion doses globally; and (ii) that vaccination rates in high-income and upper-middle-income countries are over 79 per cent, whereas the equivalent figure for low-income countries is just 26 per cent. Thus, while COVAX may be considered to have *improved* access to COVID-19 vaccines, it cannot be said to have delivered equitable access. See COVAX, 'COVAX data brief: February 2023', www.gavi.org/sites/default/files/covid/covax/COVAX-data-brief_20. pdf; Our World in Data, 'Share of people vaccinated against COVID-19,

18 April 2023', https://ourworldindata.org/explorers/coronavirus-data-explorer?zoomToSelection=true&time=2022-12-31&facet=none&pickerSort=desc&pickerMetric=population&hideControls=true&Metric=People+vaccinated+%28by+dose%29&Interval=Cumulative&Relative+to+Population=true&Color+by+test+positivity=false&country=Lower+middle+income~Upper+middle+income~High+income~Low+income

References

Anbazhagan, S. and Surekha, A. (2021) 'Nongovernmental organizations (NGOs) in global health', in R. Haring et al. (eds) *Handbook of Global Health*, Cham: Springer International Publishing, 1–11. https://doi.org/10.1007/978-3-030-05325-3_118-1

Berkley, S. (2021) 'COVAX: more than a beautiful idea', *The Lancet*, 398(10298): 388. https://doi.org/10.1016/S0140-6736(21)01544-0

Burci, G. L. (2014) 'Ebola, the Security Council and the securitization of public health', *Questions de Droit International*, 1(2).

Burci, G. L. and Eccleston-Turner, M. (2020) 'Preparing for the next pandemic: the International Health Regulations and World Health Organization during COVID-19', *Yearbook of International Disaster Law*, 2(1).

Buse, K. and Walt, G. (2002) 'The World Health Organization and global public-private health partnerships: in search of "good" global health governance', in M. R. Reich (ed.) *Public-Private Partnerships for Public Health*, Cambridge, MA: Harvard University Press, 169–195.

COVID-19 IHR Emergency Committee (no date) 'Statements', WHO. Available at: www.who.int/groups/covid-19-ihr-emergency-committee (accessed 24 April 2022).

Devi, S. (2020) 'Travel restrictions hampering COVID-19 response', *Lancet*, 395(10233): 1331–1332. https://doi.org/10.1016/S0140-6736(20)30967-3

Eccleston-Turner, M. (2023) 'WHO Processes III: Recommendation powers', in G. L. Burci, G. Le Moli and J. E. Viñuales (eds) *The International Health Regulations: Analysis and Commentary*, Oxford: Oxford University Press (Oxford Commentaries on International Law). Available at: https://papers.ssrn.com/sol3/papers.cfm?abstract_id=4620288 (accessed 7 December 2023).

Eccleston-Turner, M. and McArdle, S. (2017) 'Accountability, international law, and the World Health Organization: a need for reform?', *Global Health Governance*, XI(1): 27–40.

Eccleston-Turner, M. and McArdle, S. (2020) 'The law of responsibility and the World Health Organization: a case study on the West African Ebola outbreak', in M. Eccleston-Turner and I. Brassington (eds) *Infectious Diseases in the New Millennium: Legal and Ethical Challenges*, New York: Springer, 89–109.

Eccleston-Turner, M. and Upton, H. (2021a) 'International collaboration to ensure equitable access to vaccines for COVID-19: The ACT-Accelerator and the COVAX Facility', *The Milbank Quarterly*, 99(2): 426–449. https://doi.org/10.1111/1468-0009.12503

Eccleston-Turner, M. and Upton, H. (2021b) 'The procurement of a COVID-19 vaccine in developing countries: lessons from the 2009-H1N1 pandemic', in S. Arrowsmith, L. Butler and A. La Chimia (eds) *Public Procurement in (A) Crisis: Global Lessons from the COVID-19 Pandemic*, Oxford: Hart, 311–328.

Eccleston-Turner, M. and Villarreal, P. A. (2022) 'The World Health Organization's emergency powers: enhancing its legal and institutional accountability', *International Organizations Law Review*, 19(1): 63–89.

Eccleston-Turner, M. and Wenham, C. (2021) *Declaring a Public Health Emergency of International Concern: Between International Law and Politics*, Bristol: Bristol University Press.

Eccleston-Turner, M., McArdle, S. and Upshur, R. (2018) 'Inter-institutional relationships in global health: regulating coordination and ensuring accountability', *Global Health Governance*, XII(2): 83–99.

Fidler, D. P. (2005) 'From international sanitary conventions to global health security: the new International Health Regulations', *Chinese Journal of International Law*, 4(2): 325–392. https://doi.org/10.1093/chinesejil/jmi029

Fidler, D. P. and Gostin, L. O. (2006) 'The new International Health Regulations: an historic development for international law and public health', *The Journal of Law, Medicine & Ethics*, 34(1): 85–94. https://doi.org/10.1111/j.1748-720X.2006.00011.x

Gavi (2020) 'The COVAX Facility: global procurement for COVID-19 vaccines'. Available at: www.gavi.org/sites/default/files/covid/The-COVAX-Facility_backgrounder-3.pdf (accessed 7 August 2020).

Gavi (no date) 'COVAX vaccine rollout: country updates'. Available at: www.gavi.org/covax-vaccine-roll-out (accessed 16 July 2021).

Gostin, L. and Friedman, E. (2014) 'Ebola: a crisis in global health leadership', *The Lancet*, 384(9951): 1323–1325.

Gostin, L. and Mok, E. (2009) 'Grand challenges in global health governance', *British Medical Bulletin*, 90(1): 7–18. https://doi.org/10.1093/bmb/ldp014

Gostin, L. et al. (2019) 'Ebola in the Democratic Republic of the Congo: time to sound a global alert?', *The Lancet*, 393(10172): 617–620. https://doi.org/10.1016/S0140-6736(19)30243-0

Gostin, L., Moon, S. and Mason Meier, B. (2020) 'Reimagining global health governance in the age of COVID-19', *American Journal of Public Health*, 110(11): 1615–1619.

GOV.UK (2021) 'UK marks one year since deploying world's first COVID-19 vaccine', GOV.UK, 8 December. Available at: www.gov.uk/government/news/uk-marks-one-year-since-deploying-worlds-first-covid-19-vaccine (accessed 31 May 2022).

Grogan, J. (2022) 'COVID-19, the rule of law and democracy: analysis of legal responses to a global health crisis', *Hague Journal on the Rule of Law*, 14(2–3): 349–369. https://doi.org/10.1007/s40803-022-00168-8

Habibi, R. et al. (2020) 'Do not violate the International Health Regulations during the COVID-19 outbreak', *The Lancet*, 395(10225): 664–666. https://doi.org/10.1016/S0140-6736(20)30373-1

Hampton, A., Upton, H. and Eccleston-Turner, M. (2021) 'The WHO's procurement of pandemic vaccines: private law by a public body', in S. McArdle and S. Swizter (eds) *Elgar Companion to the Law and Practice of the World Health Organization*, Cheltenham: Edward Elgar (in press).

Heymann, D. L. and Roider, G. (2004) 'SARS: a global response to an international threat', *The Brown Journal of World Affairs*, 10(2): 185–197.

Kamradt-Scott, A. (2010) 'The WHO Secretariat, norm entrepreneurship, and global disease outbreak control', *Journal of International Organizations Studies*, 1(1): 72–89.

Kamradt-Scott, A. (2015) *Managing Global Health Security: The World Health Organization and Disease Outbreak Control*, Basingstoke: Palgrave Macmillan.

Kiernan, S., DeVita, M. and Bollyky, J. (2020) 'Tracking coronavirus in countries with and without travel bans', *Think Global Health*, 7 April. Available at: www.thinkglobalhealth.org/article/tracking-coronavirus-countries-and-without-travel-bans (accessed 4 June 2021).

Larinova, M. and Kirton, J. (2020) 'Global governance after the COVID-19 crisis', *International Organisations Research Journal*, 15(2): 7–17.

Lee, K. and Kamradt-Scott, A. (2014) 'The multiple meanings of global health governance: a call for conceptual clarity', *Globalization and Health*, 10(1): 28. https://doi.org/10.1186/1744-8603-10-28

Lisk, F. and Šehović, A. B. (2020) 'Rethinking global health governance in a changing world order for achieving sustainable development: the role and potential of the "rising powers"', *Fudan Journal of the Humanities and Social Sciences*, 13(1): 45–65. https://doi.org/10.1007/s40647-018-00250-2

Mackey, T. K. (2016) 'The Ebola outbreak: catalyzing a "shift" in global health governance?', *BMC Infectious Diseases*, 16(1): 699. https://doi.org/10.1186/s12879-016-2016-y

Mason Meier, B. et al. (2022) 'Travel restrictions and variants of concern: global health laws need to reflect evidence', *Bulletin of the World Health Organization*, 100(03): 178–178A. https://doi.org/10.2471/BLT.21.287735

Meier, B. M., Habibi, R. and Yang, Y. T. (2020) 'Travel restrictions violate international law', *Science*, 367(6485): 1436. https://doi.org/10.1126/science.abb6950

Partridge, J. and Kieny, M. P. (2010) 'Global production of seasonal and pandemic (H1N1) influenza vaccines in 2009–2010 and comparison with previous estimates and global action plan targets', *Vaccine*, 28(30): 4709–4712. https://doi.org/10.1016/j.vaccine.2010.04.083

Storey, A. and Eccleston-Turner, M. (2022) 'Transparency, accountability, and legitimacy within the UN Universal Periodic Review', in S. Santino, F. Regilme and I. Hadiprayitno (eds) *Human Rights at Risk: Rethinking International Institutions, American Power, and the Future of Dignity*, New Brunswick, NJ: Rutgers University Press, 25–39.

Syam, N. and Alas, M. (2021) 'Strengthening WHO for future health emergencies while battling COVID-19: major outcomes of the 2021 World Health Assembly', *South Centre Policy Brief*, 106.

Tejpar, A. and Hoffman, S. J. (2017) 'Canada's violation of international law during the 2014–16 Ebola outbreak', *Canadian Yearbook of International Law/Annuaire canadien de droit international*, 54: 366–383. https://doi.org/10.1017/cyl.2017.18

UN (United Nations) (2020) 'Independent Oversight and Advisory Committee for the WHO Health Emergencies Programme, Statement to the 73rd World Health Assembly', UN Doc A73/10. Available at: https://cdn.who.int/media/docs/default-source/dco/independent-oversight-and-advisory-committee/a73_10-en-ioac-report1cc3d833-6979-4ac3-a0ea-21b4a6bf1670.pdf?sfvrsn=d2bcf955_1&download=true (accessed 31 May 2022).

UN (United Nations) (2016) 'Reform of WHO's work in health emergency management: WHO Health Emergencies Programme', Report by WHO Director-General Margret Chan to the 69th WHA, 5 May 2016, UN Doc A69/30.

Wenham, C. (2017) 'What we have learnt about the World Health Organization from the Ebola outbreak', *Philosophical Transactions of the Royal Society B: Biological Sciences*, 372(1721): 20160307. https://doi.org/10.1098/rstb.2016.0307

Wenham, C. et al. (2021) 'Problems with traffic light approaches to public health emergencies of international concern', *The Lancet*, 397(10287): 1856–1858. https://doi.org/10.1016/S0140-6736(21)00474-8

WHO (1948) 'Constitution of the World Health Organization', 14 UNTS 185. Available at: https://apps.who.int/gb/bd/PDF/bd47/EN/constitution-en.pdf (accessed 7 December 2023).

WHO (2005) 'International Health Regulations', UNTS 2509. Available at: https://iris.who.int/bitstream/handle/10665/246107/9789241580496-eng.pdf?sequence=1 (accessed 7 December 2023).

WHO (2011) 'Main operational lessons learnt from the WHO Pandemic Influenza A (H1N1) Vaccine Deployment Initiative', report of a WHO meeting held in Geneva, Switzerland, 13–15 December 2010, Geneva: World Health Organization. Available at: http://apps.who.int/iris/bitstream/10665/44711/1/9789241564342_eng.pdf (accessed 12 June 2020).

WHO (2013) 'WHO's role in global health governance', Report by the Director-General, EB132/5 Add.5, 18 January 2013, Provisional agenda item 5, Geneva: World Health Organization. Available at: https://apps.who.int/gb/ebwha/pdf_files/EB132/B132_5Add5-en.pdf (accessed 18 May 2022).

WHO (2020) 'Statement on the Second Meeting of the International Health Regulations (2005) Emergency Committee regarding the coronavirus disease (COVID-19) pandemic'. Available at: www.who.int/news/item/30-01-2020-statement-on-the-second-meeting-of-the-international-health-regulations-(2005)-emergency-committee-regarding-the-outbreak-of-novel-coronavirus-(2019-ncov) (accessed 8 June 2021).

WHO (2021) 'COVID-19 vaccine doses shipped by the COVAX Facility head to Ghana, marking beginning of global rollout', World Health Organization, 24 February. Available at: www.who.int/news/item/24-02-2021-covid-19-vaccine-doses-shipped-by-the-covax-facility-head-to-ghana-marking-beginning-of-global-rollout (accessed 31 May 2022).

WHO (no date) 'Statement on the meeting of the International Health Regulations (2005) Emergency Committee for Ebola virus disease in the Democratic Republic of the Congo on 14 June 2019'. Available at: www.who.int/news-room/detail/14-06-2019-statement-on-the-meeting-of-the-international-health-regulations-(2005)-emergency-committee-for-ebola-virus-disease-in-the-democratic-republic-of-the-congo (accessed 19 March 2020).

Yach, D. (2016) 'World Health Organization reform: a normative or an operational organization?', *American Journal of Public Health*, 106(11): 1904–1906. https://doi.org/10.2105/AJPH.2016.303376

Index

Entries in **bold** refer to tables; entries in *italics* refer to figures. References of the form "XnY" refer to note Y on page X.

Access to COVID-19 Tools (ACT) Accelerator 180
accountability 4, 49
 in data ethics 84
 as ethical principle 77
 and ethical values 131
 and global health governance 173, 175–7, 181–5
 and public engagement 141
 in social care 64–6, 69
Ada Lovelace Institute 150, 162, 164, 166
adult-centrism 109
Adult Social Care Outcomes Framework (ASCOF) 62–4, 68
Adult Social Care Survey 64
advance purchase agreements (APAs) 181–3
advenants 22–4
Aebischer, Pascale 5
agency 43, 62, 65, 151, 155, 163
agenda day method 95, 102–9
Agenda for Sustainable Development 110
AIDS epidemic 15
allocation problems 58
ambivalence 159, 164

Arnstein, Sherry 124, 127
artificial intelligence 94
Arts and Humanities Research Council (AHRC) xii, 94
authority to act, co-producing 87–9
autonomy, and relationships 43–4

behavioural fatigue 127
Bingham Centre for the Rule of Law 150, 162–4, 166
Black, Asian and Minority Ethnic people 56, 66, 98, 116n5, 134
Brazil 141
Burall, Simon 139
burnout xix, 46
Burton, Jenny 60

Callard, Felicity 14, 16
Camden Council 139–40
Capacity Tracker 58, 63, 66, 82
care
 in care homes 70
 and infection prevention 30, 39
 markers of 44
 as value 64–5

care homes xv, xix, 7
  data on 56–61, 65–6, 70–1,
    75, 82–3
  deaths in 54–5, 59–60
  protective ring around 81–2, 87
  staff vaccinations in 63, 129
Challenge Trials 78
Chatham House Rules 143n12
child- and youth-led
    organisations 112
child facilitators 102, 105, 107
children
  acting on views of 113
  engaging with 111–13
  impact of COVID-19 response
    on 97–100
  lack of focus on 101
  participation in decision-
    making 109–11
  speaking for themselves 101–2
  vaccination of 130
  views on COVID-19 response
    94–6, 102–9, 113–14
Children's Commissioners 113
children's rights 8, 96
Children's Rights Impact
    Assessments 109–10
China 176
cholera 160, 162
Citizens' Assemblies 126, 140
Citizens' Juries 9, 126, 150–1, 153,
    162–4, 166–7
civil liberties 8, 88, 157
Coalition for Epidemic Preparedness
    Innovation (CEPI) 181
collective dialogue, real-time 151
collective stories 26
Committee on Standards in Public
    Life 138
commonality 22, 26
common-sense philosophy 127
comorbidities 56, 130
competence, reputations of 139
confidence, crises of 168
Conservative Party 84, 87,
    131–2, 141

consultation documents
    111, 116n15
contact tracing
  data generated by 161
  engagement with 127
  removal of requirements
    for 83
  and surveillance 155–7
contact tracing apps 80, 83,
    85–6, 126
  see also NHS Test and Trace
contemporaneity 24–6
Control of Patient Information
    (COPI) 80–1, 83–4, 86
Cooper, Fred 1–2
co-presence 24, 26
CoRAY Project 126
Coronavirus Research Centre
    (CRC) 162
Councils with Adult Social
    Services Responsibilities
    (CASSRs) 62
COVAX Facility 173–4, 179,
    181–5, 185n4
COVID-19 pandemic
  acceptable risks in 78
  arts and humanities research
    during xii–xxii, 1–2, 6
  care infrastructure in 63
  and children's rights 100
  decision making in 3–5,
    9–10, 65
  declaring an end to 83–4, 88
  impact on democracy 150–3
  and inequalities 66
  infection prevention and care in
    29–30, 32, 46
  life before 23
  and policy dynamism 50
  reconfiguration of possibility 21
  and relationships 36–7
  temporality of 14–15
  use of data in 56, 79–81, 88
critical workers 98, 115n4
cronyism 131
Cummings, Dominic 154–5

data
    and authority to act 87–8
    creating vulnerabilities 86–7
    quality of 159–60
Data Charter 139–40
data collection xvi, 80–1
    and contact tracing 156
    end of 89
    ethical evaluations of 86
    online 105
    in social care 64, 66
    via technology 168n1
data consent systems 70
data-driven decision-making 8–9, 94–5
    children's views on 103, 107–8
    impact on children 96–7, 99, 101–2, 113–15
    and UKGDPR 106
data episodes 79–84, 87
data ethics 7–8, 77, 84–5, 87, 89
datafication of children 96, 101
data governance 66–7
data infrastructures 54–5, 57–8
    and democracy 85
    for social care 55, 60–7, 69, 82
data not dates approach 94
data pandemic 79–81
data protection 101, 156
Data Saves Lives 67–8
data sharing 86, 96–7, 107–8
data sources
    multiple 81
    novel 60
data use 7–8
    ethical 78
dataveillance 101, 114
death 2
    visibility of 19
decentralised logics 65
decision-making
    academic influence on 135
    citizen participation in 141
    and data infrastructures 57
    emergency 151
    ethical tensions of 137
    long-term structures of 139
    pandemic-specific approaches 32, 50–1
    public engagement in 124
    public involvement in 35
    and relationships 30–1, 37, 43–4, 46–7, **48**
    self-mythologised model of 129
    values informing 33, 131, 133, 159
    see also data-driven decision-making
deliberation, institutionalising 166, 168
deliberative approaches 126, 140
deliberative engagement 125
democracy
    core principles of 150
    pausing 150–2, 166
    and quality of science 159–60
democratic nation-states 8–9, 150–1, 153–4, 161, 164, 167–8
democratic spaces 3
denominator problem 57–60
Dewey, John 127
digital infrastructures 58
digital platforms, age-appropriate 112
disease 14
    aetiological framework of 18–19
drama, epidemics as 12–14, 16–17, 20, 26
dynamism 50

Ebola 173, 178–80
educational inequalities 98
electronic relationships 36–7
emergence, of epidemics 16–17, 19, 27n2
Emergency Committee 178–9
emergency data ethics 8, 89
emergency powers
    and data use 7
    ending 86
    and the social contract 151–2

emergency powers (*continued*)
    UK use of 3–4
    WHO use of 9, 177–8, 184
    see also state of emergency
Emerging Minds 126
endemic disease 13–14, 16, 26
end of life 34, 38
en-present-ment 25
epidemicity 17–20, 22, 24–5
epidemics
    as extraordinary events 17–18
    as life-event 20–4
    literary form of 6, 12–17
    as nested 24–6
    visualising 19–20
epistemic authority 184
epistemic framings xxv, 5
epistemic power 59
epistemological pluralism 159, 161–2, 165–6
equitable access to vaccines 181–5, 185n4
ethical analysis 69, 132
ethical challenges 6, 29–30, 33–5, 45, 47, 131–2
ethical deliberations 125, 142
ethical expertise 136–7
ethical frameworks 32, 47, 85–6
ethical perspectives 140, 142n1
ethical principles 77–8
ethical unit of analysis 64
ethical values
    in decision-making **48–9**, 131–2, 134, 136–7, 142
    in maternity and paediatric care 32–4
ethics 2
    relational 44
ethics advice 10, 84–5
Ethics Advisory Group to NHSX 77, 90n1
ethics washing 84–5, 89
European Citizens' Panels (ECPs) 140

European Convention on Human Rights (ECHR) 98, 116n6
European Union, Conference on the Future of Europe 140
event, senses of 17–24, 26
event-ness 24
events, interpretative function of 23
events and conferences 111–12
everyday life xxiii, 12, 85
extraordinariness 17–18

Fair Allocation Framework 182
fairness 49–50, 77, 84, 86
Fitzgerald, Des 1
focus groups 33–5, 39, 45
    for children 112
    on public engagement 125, 129
freedom-loving 127, 142n3
freedom of movement 79, 158, 163
freedoms, personal 87, 130, 165
free school meals 96
future, evential 22–4

Gavi the Vaccine Alliance 181–4
Geidt, Christopher 138
General Practice Data for Planning and Research 163
Gibson, Michael 54–6
global health governance (GHG) 9, 172, 174–7
Goldacre Report 67–9
good governance 4, 9, 168, 185
    and accountability 69
    citizens' juries and 163–4
    during the pandemic 150, 153
    and international organisations 173–4
    principles of 4, 150, 164, 167, 184
    of technologies 164, **165**
    see also global health governance
governance shift 181
Gray, Sue 84, 155
Greene, Jeremy 15
green space, public 116n5

H1N1 Influenza pandemic 183–4
Hancock, Matt 81–2
hard-to-reach children 112
Harris, Donald 54–6
Health and Care Act 2022 68
healthcare policy, relational approach to 47
healthcare professionals xviii–xix
  ability to care 7, 29–31
  and moral distress 34
  relationship with patients 40–2
  safety of 46
  and senior decision-makers 33, 38–9
  working from home 40
Health Data Research UK 126
health emergencies
  principles for decision-making **165**
  WHO and 172–4, 177–9, 184
Healy, Margaret 19
HEPI (Higher Education Policy Institute) xiii
hermeneutics 21, 26
Hobbes, Thomas 152
home-schooled children xvi, 111
home working 133
Hopkins Van Mil (HVM) 131–6, 140
House of Lords 4, 140–1
human connections xxv, 2, 65
human rights xviii, 167–8
  and children's rights 100, 114
  and surveillance 77
human stories 1

Iceland 141
illiberal democracies 150
illness time 15
immediacy xx, 23
Independent Commission on UK Public Health Emergency Powers 4
Independent Oversight and Advisory Committee (IOAC) 180
Index of Multiple Deprivation (IMD) 103
infection prevention 2, 6–7
  and care 29–30
  impact on relationships 40–1, 44, 46
infectiousness 13, 19, 21
information flow, one-way 128, 143n5
information governance 56, 60, 66–7
informing decisions 94, 136
Institute for Government Timeline 78–9
institutional approaches 43
Integrated Care Systems 68
intelligibility 13, 20, 23
International Health Regulations 173, 176–9, 184
international law 173, 184
international organisations 9, 174–5, 184
Investing in Children 8, 95, 102
invisibility 89
Israel 154

Jacobellis v. Ohio 175
Johns Hopkins data dashboard 161–2
Johnson, Boris 1–3, 79, 84, 87–8, 131
Joint Council of Vaccination and Immunisation (JCVI) 130
justice xix, xxvii
  crossgenerational xiii
  as ethical principle 77

Keller, Richard 15
key workers xviii, 2, 97
knowledge
  deep 138
  proposition and performative 136

Lachenal, Guillaume 15
large hospitals, collaboration within 36
leadership, physically remote 37
learning disabilities 60
legitimacy
 and deliberative processes 144n15, 153, 167
 and democratic principles 150
 and global health governance 174–5, 177, 185
legitimacy to act 87–8
liberal democracies 150, 152–4
life-events 6, 16, 20–6
life-stories 26
lived experience xxii, 17
lockdowns
 children in 97–9
 decision-making on 8, 101
 democracy in 150–1
 in the UK 2, 33, 79–80, 83–4, 127
logic
 dramaturgic 12, 14
 relational 43
long COVID xix, 14–15, 21–2, 134

Magnus, Laurie 138
management, top-down 68
market-oriented logics 65
masks 36
 children's views on 105, 109
maternity and paediatric services 29–33, 35–42
 family in 44–5
Maternity Voices Partnership (MVP) 35, 51n4
ME/CFS (Myalgic Encephalomyelitis/Chronic Fatigue Syndrome) 14
mental health xiii, 98, 134
Moral and Ethical Advisory Group (MEAG) 138
moral distress 31, 34, 46, 51n3
morbidity xvii, 14, 18–19

mortality 14, 18–19, 60
mutual aid 36, 46

narratives xxv–xxvi, 12, 56, 124
National Audit Office (NAO) 156–7
National Health Service 6
 capacity to treat children 98
 contact tracing by 80, 85, 90n1, 97, 105
  see also NHS Test and Trace
 convergence of systems and services 68
 data systems 58–9
 digital arm of see NHSX
 discharge decisions 57
 maternity and paediatric services in 29, 31–3
 priority to protect 82
 staff safety 45
neglect 89
NHS see National Health Service
NHS COVID Data Store 81
NHS Test and Trace 67, 99, 105, 156–7
NHSX 77, 80
Nicholas, Rachael 5
9/11 terrorist attacks 86
Nolan Principles of Public Life 85, 138
non-discrimination 98–9, 111, 165
non-government organisations (NGOs) 113, 139, 172
non-maleficence 77
Northumbria University 94, 103

Observatory for Monitoring Data-Driven Approaches to COVID-19 (OMDDAC) 94–6, 102–4, 108–11, 113
Office of National Statistics (ONS) 81–2
Office of Qualifications and Examinations Regulation (OFQUAL) 99, 116n7
online engagement xiv, 104

opacity 131
open society 159–60, 162, 166
organisational rules 47
Organisation for Economic and Cultural Development (OECD) 125, 144n15
overreach 9, 151, 167
over-surveillance 65, 86

Palantir 81
Pandemic and Beyond series xii, xiv–xvii, xxi–xxvi, xxviin2, 5
pandemic ethics 133, 137
Pandemic Influenza Ethical Framework 85
Pandemic Influenza Preparedness Framework 173
pandemic rules 3, 56
pandemics, definition of 27n1
pandemic time xix, 51
participation
  ladder of 124, 129–30, 132, 140–1
  Lundy's model of 110–11, 113
participatory budgeting 141
participatory democracy 139, 141
participatory engagement 135, 142, 143n5
participatory governance 125, 139–40
participatory infrastructures 9, 151, 167
participatory turn 167
partnership, in citizen participation 129
Partygate scandal 4, 84, 88, 131, 143n7
Patel, Reema 10n2
Patient and Public Involvement (PPI) 35
patient relationships 40–1
Pelling, Margaret 13
people-in-relationships 44
performative language 19
personal data 96
personal fulfilment xxv, 2

personal protective equipment (PPE) xv, 37, 40, 59, 82, 87
  allocation decisions 59, 63
  and maternity care 30, 37–8, 40, 45
  procurement scandals 67
PHEIC (Public Health Emergency of International Concern) 17, 27n2, 178–9
phenomenological theory 17
plague writing 19, 25
police, access to COVID-19 data 103, 107–8, 155
policymaking
  and epistemological pluralism 159, 162, 166
  ethical influence over 134, 136, 138–9
  impact on those affected 132
  informing 129
  pandemic 135–6
  publics involved in 124–5, 134, 142
Popper, Karl 159, 162
Porto Alegre 141
possibility, reconfiguration of 18, 21–2
poverty xix, 7, 98, 134
PPE *see* personal protective equipment
privacy
  of children 99
  and contact tracing 80–1, 155–7
  as ethical principle 77
  and public health 86
  violation of 63, 66
psychologists, support for healthcare professionals 34, 42
public dialogue 125, 132–3, 135, 140, 142
public engagement 8–9, 124
  ethical analysis of 132
  inadequacies in UK government 126–9, 131
  institutionalised 141

public engagement (*continued*)
  in the pandemic 125–6
  role of xxv, 5
public ethics 138
public health xxv, 2
  in decision-making 5–6, 130
  red lines for 166
public involvement 35, 134, 137
Public-Private-Partnership (PPP) 172, 181, 185
publics 8
  informing and influencing 127
  perspectives of 124–5, 139–40
  in UK decision-making 129–30
  use of term 142n1
public values 125, 132–3, 139–40, 142n1

QCovid algorithm 97

racism xix
rationality, and relationality 43–4
Rawls, John 152
red lines 164, 166
regulatory frameworks 64, 125, 163
relational agents 43
relationality 7, 31–2, 43–7, 49
relational processes 51n8
relational values 65
relationships
  damage caused to 40–1
  enactment of 50
  in healthcare decision-making **48–9**
  in maternity care 7, 30–3, 35–42
  networks of 42–5
  risks of disrupting 45–7
Renaissance, plague writing of 19
representativeness 104, 132
research ethics 78
Reset Ethics project 29, 31–3, 51
responsibility
  as ethical principle 77
  in relational ethics 44
rights-based approaches 89

risk aversion 78
Romano, Claude 18, 21–2, 24–6
Rosenberg, Charles 12–15, 19, 23, 26
Rourke, Elizabeth 21, 23
Rousseau, Jean-Jacques 152
rule of law xxv, 2, 9, 150, 167–8
  abrogation of 154–5
  citizens' juries and 163–4

SARS (severe acute respiratory syndrome) 172–3
SARS-CoV-2 *see* COVID-19 pandemic
school closures 8, 95, 97–8, 101, 105, 109, 115
school grades, algorithmic determination of 103–4, 107
"the science" xxv, 1, 6, 124, 129
science-led approach 159, 161–2
Scientific Advisory Group for Emergencies (SAGE) 130
scientisation 167
scientism 159
Scottish government 126
selfhood, past and current 25
self-isolation 8, 83, 94
  police monitoring of 103–4, 108
senior decision-makers 33, 37–8, 46
shame 2–3
Shielded Patients List 163
Singapore 155
Slack, Paul 13
Smallman, Melanie 65
Snow, John 160–1
Snowden, Frank 12
social care xiv, 7
  complexity of 61–3, 67
  data infrastructure for 54–5, 82
  data policy for 67–9
  ethical issues in 138
  missing data for 56–60, 87
  multiple scales of 65–7
  values of 63–5
  what data measures in 69–71

Social Care White Paper 2021 68
social contract 151–3, 155
social distancing xv, 8
  impact on children of 98
  and interviews with children 102, 104
  and maternity care 34, 41–2, 45
social distancing rules 30, 45, 127
social groupings xxv, 2
social media
  children's use of 101, 106
  and data pandemic 79
  recruitment to focus groups on 35
solidarity 137, 143n13, 174
Spiegelhalter, David 114
state of emergency 8, 150–1, 153–4
Steel, David 13
stigma 3
Sunak, Rishi 138
sunset clauses 166
surveillance 60, 66, 89
  and democracy 154–6
  and ethical principles 77–8
  and vaccine passports 158
  wastewater testing as 104
surveillance infrastructure 85
Swiss cheese model 143n10
syndemic 99
system performativity 62–3

Taiwan 140
technologies, rapid acceleration of 155
temporality xix, 14–16, 22, 25–6
Temporary Recommendations 176, 178
test and trace 83, 85, 88
Thomas, Gaëtan 15
tokenism 127, 129
Tony Blair Institute for Global Change 158
transparency
  in data ethics 84
  in emergency contexts 89
  as ethical principle 77
  and global health governance 175–7, 181, 185
  lack of 37, 85, 156, 176–7, 183–4
  and public engagement 132, 134–5, 141
transparent communication 38
travel restrictions 105, 172, 176
trust
  and contact tracing 157
  and global health governance 174–6
  and transparency 134–5
trusted research environments (TREs) 69
trustworthiness 141, 153, 165
Twain, Mark 160

UK see United Kingdom
underfunding, chronic 180
under-surveillance 86
United Kingdom
  care outside hospitals 61
  contact tracing in 156–7
  COVID-19 response in xvii–xix, 1–4, 33
  data and COVID-19 in 78–84
  Data Ethics Framework 84
  data infrastructures in 57
  deliberative events in 133
  emergency powers in 151, 154
  lifting restrictions in 20, 129–31
  lockdowns in 97–8
  participatory governance in 140
  research funding in xxi
  self-isolation rules in 29
  social care sector in 54–5, 59, 70–1
  temporary data measures in 66–7
  vaccine passports in 157–8
United Kingdom General Data Protection Regulation (UKGDPR) 106–7

United Kingdom Pandemic Ethics Accelerator 125, 131–2, 134, 137–9, 142
United Kingdom Research and Innovation (UKRI) xiv, xvi–xvii, xxviin2, 137
United Nations Convention on the Rights of the Child (UNCRC) 96, 98–100, 106, 110–11, 114–15, 115n2, 116n6

vaccine certification 127, 137, 157–8
Vaccine Deployment Initiative (VDI) 183–4
vaccine mandates 129
vaccine nationalism 174
vaccine passports 157–8, 161, 163, 166
vaccine procurement 182
value-free policymaking 129–31
value judgements 63–4, 140
Vargha, Dora 15
voices, missing 8
vulnerabilities xiii, xxiv, 26
  creating 82, 86–7
vulnerable children 97–8

wastewater testing 103–5, 107
wave graph 19
welfare state 7, 61, 87
Westminster policy workshop 134–9
WHO *see* World Health Organization
working practices, changed 7, 29, 33–4, 40, 42
World Health Organization (WHO) xviii, xxv, 5, 9, 172–3
  good governance of 177–8
  Guidance for Managing Ethical Issues in Infectious Disease 78
  Health Emergencies programme (WHE) 179–81, 185
  on pandemics 27n1
  trust and legitimacy of 174–7, 184–5
World Medical Association 78

Zoom 1, 36, 41, 102

EU authorised representative for GPSR:
Easy Access System Europe, Mustamäe tee 50,
10621 Tallinn, Estonia
gpsr.requests@easproject.com

www.ingramcontent.com/pod-product-compliance
Ingram Content Group UK Ltd.
Pitfield, Milton Keynes, MK11 3LW, UK
UKHW021823140426
5217IPUK00004B/66